Sirtfood Diet

3 Books In 1: The Complete Cookbook For Beginners To Boost Metabolism, Lose Weight And Get Lean Quickly With 250 Healthy, Delicious, And Tasty Recipes, Including A 4 Weeks Meal Plan

Sirtfood Diet for Beginners

Table of Contents

Introduction 1
Chapter One: Sirtuins Studies 7
Chapter Two: Fighting Fat 9
Chapter Three: The Wonders Of Well-Being 12
Chapter Four: Types Of Sirtfoods 13
Chapter Five: Building A Healthy Diet That Works 15
Chapter Six: Top 20 Sirtfoods 20
Chapter Seven: Phase 1: Losing 7 Pounds In Seven Days 26
Chapter Eight: Phase 2: Maintenance 31
Chapter Nine: Sirtfoods For Life 33
Chapter Ten: Frequently Asked Questions And Answers 39

INTRODUCTION

Racheal felt her world crumbling when she heard the word emanating from the mouth of her doctor. She had given up work a few months earlier at just fifty-one and was eagerly planning her next life adventures. She had just been reunited with her early-life sweetheart, Charles, after being apart for thirty years, in what could have graced a Hollywood romance script. They would marry soon. She was then told that she had breast cancer. Luckily the treatment was a success, but the chemotherapy side effects took their toll. Racheal has always struggled with her weight over the years and has tried every diet trend going, only to regain the weight plus more every time. But she has just not felt good now. She felt "uncomfortable, heavy, and lethargic." She fell into a pattern of comfort eating, and she felt like she had to complete a marathon with the simplest of activities she used to enjoy, like going out for a walk. Racheal had gained 20 pounds in just a matter of months. The doctor then informed her that she would spend the next ten years on anticancer medication. It was the popular tamoxifen drug, well-known for causing weight gain and lethargy. She was confronted with the prospect of swallowing a tablet daily to stave off cancer, but at the expense of her vitality and feeling good about her.

Still, Racheal had decided not to let her beat it. Her now-husband, Charles, was a cynical eater, being the rock by her side. But he had little to lose after reading about a new weight-loss diet focused on the power of consuming natural plant foods that boasted enormous health benefits. They embarked on the Sirtfood Diet, together. Racheal lost 20 kilos within the first six weeks. Charles had lost 12 pounds himself, despite not carrying much excess weight to start with. To Racheal, this was a big breakthrough, but the change of how she felt was much bigger. Her confidence levels soared and returned to her zest for life. The need for comfort-eating disappeared, and the appeal of junk food was lost. She was back to her normal activities again, and she felt better and better with each passing day. In Racheal's words, "It's one of the best things that we've ever done, the best that we've both felt in years. This is not a diet in the usual sense but a way of eating for life. I don't feel the side effects of the medication now, and I never have to worry about getting 'dieted' again."

For the hundreds of millions who this year will follow popularized diets, fewer than 1 percent will experience substantial weight loss. Not only will they be fighting to make a difference in the bulge war, but they are doing little to stem the wave of chronic disease that has ravaged modern society.

We can live longer but have no safer lives. Stunningly, in just ten years, the amount of time we spend in ill health has doubled from 20 to 40 percent. It means that we are spending almost 32 years of our lives now in poor health. Just check the stats here. One in ten is suffering from diabetes right now, and three are on the verge of having it. Two out of every five people are diagnosed with cancer at some point in their lives. If you see three women over 50, one of them may have an osteoporotic fracture. If it takes you to read a single page of this book in the average time, a new case of Alzheimer's is going to arise, and someone is going to die of heart failure — and that's just in the USA.

For those reasons, "Dieting" was never our thing. That's until we discovered Sirtfoods, a revolutionary new — and easy — way to eat your way to weight loss and great health.

What Are Sirtfoods?

The moment we cut back on calories, we trigger an energy shortage, known as the "skinny gene," causing a raft of positive changes. It puts the body in a kind of survival mode where fat is prevented from processing, and normal processes of growth are put on hold. Instead, the body turns its attention to burning up its fat reserves and flipping on powerful housekeeping genes that repair and rejuvenate our cells, effectively giving them a clean spring. The upshot is weight loss, and increased susceptibility to disease.

But, as many dieters are aware, cutting calories comes at a cost. Reducing short-term energy consumption induces hunger, irritability, tiredness, and muscle weakness. Long-term calorie restriction is causing our metabolism to stagnate. This is the downfall of all calorie-restrictive diets and paves the way back on the weight for a piling up. Ninety-nine percent of dietitians are doomed to a long-term failure for these reasons.

All of this has led us to ask a big question: can our thin gene be enabled with all the great benefits that bring and all those disadvantages without having to hold to an extreme calorie constraint?

It's time to join Sirtfoods, a collection of newly discovered wonder-foods. Sirtfoods are especially rich in special nutrients that can activate in our bodies the same slim genes when we eat them as the calorie restriction does. Such genes come to be called sirtuins. They first came to light in a pioneering study in 2003 when researchers discovered that resveratrol, a compound found in red grape skin and red wine, greatly increased the life span of the yeast. Interestingly, resveratrol had the same effect on longevity as calorie restriction, but this was accomplished without reducing energy intake. Resveratrol has also been shown to be able to extend the lifetime of worms, insects, fish, and even honeybees. Early-stage experiments from mice to humans suggest that resveratrol protects against the adverse effects of high-calorie, high-fat, and high-sugar diets; encourages healthy aging by slowing age-related diseases, and improves fitness.

Ultimately, it has been shown to imitate the effects of calorie restriction.

Red wine, with its rich resveratrol content, was hailed as the original sirtfood, describing the health benefits associated with its consumption and also why people who drink red wine gain less weight.

Upon the discovery of resveratrol, the field of health science was at the cusp of something significant, and the pharmaceutical industry wasted no time jumping on board. Researchers began screening thousands of various chemicals for their ability to activate our sirtuin genes. That revealed a number of natural plant compounds, not just resveratrol, with significant sirtuin-activating properties. It was also found that a given food could contain a whole range of these plant compounds, which could work together to help both absorb and optimize the food's sirtuin-activating effect. It had been one of the big mysteries concerning resveratrol. Resveratrol testing scientists also had to use much higher doses to provide a benefit than we realize when drunk as part of the red wine. Nevertheless, as well as resveratrol, red wine contains a range of other natural plant compounds, including high amounts of piceatannol as well as quercetin, myricetin, and epicatechin, each of which has been shown to independently activate our sirtuin genes and, more importantly, to work in coordination.

The dilemma for the pharmaceutical industry is that they are unable to sell the next major breakthrough product as a nutrient or food category. Instead, hundreds of millions of dollars were invested in the hopes of uncovering a Shangri-la pill to develop and test synthetic compounds. There are currently multiple studies of sirtuin-activating drugs for a multitude of chronic diseases, as well as the first-ever FDA-approved trial to investigate whether the medicine can slow aging.

If history has taught us something, it's that we shouldn't hold as much hope for this synthetic ambrosia as it might be as tantalizing. The pharmaceutical and wellness industries have continually tried to replicate the effects of extracted nutrients and drugs from foods and diets. Yet, time and again, it has come up short. Why wait ten more years for the acceptance of these so-called wonder medications and the possible side effects they bring, when right now we have all the amazing benefits available from the food we eat at our fingertips?

So as the pharmaceutical industry relentlessly chases a drug-like silver bullet, we need to retrain our focus on dieting. And at the same time, those efforts were underway; the world of nutritional science was also evolving, raising some of its own big questions. Besides red wine, were there other high-level foods that were able to activate our sirtuin genes from these unique nutrients? And if so, what were their effects on triggering fat loss and fighting disease?

Not All Fruits and Vegetables Are Equal

Researchers at Harvard University have performed two of the largest nutritional studies in U.S. history since 1986: the Health Professionals Follow-Up Study, which explores men's eating patterns and well-being, and the Nurses' Health Report, which investigates the same for women. Based on this vast wealth of data, researchers examined the correlation between more than 124,000 people's dietary habits and changes in body weight over a 24-year period ending in 2011.

Something interesting they noted. Consumption of such plant foods as part of a typical American diet stayed off weight gain, but eating others had no effect whatsoever. How distinct were they from each other? It all boiled down to whether certain types of naturally occurring plant chemicals known as polyphenols made the food rich. Almost every one of us continues putting on weight as we age, but the consumption of higher polyphenol concentrations had a major impact on preventing this. When studied in greater depth, only some forms of polyphenols stood out as being effective in keeping people lean, the researchers found. Among those effective were the same groups of natural plant chemicals which the pharmaceutical industry was furiously trying to turn into a wonder pill for their ability to turn on our sirtuin genes.

The result was profound: Not all plant foods (including fruits and vegetables) are equal when it comes to managing our weight. Instead, we need to start studying plant foods for their polyphenol content and then look into their ability to turn on our "skinny" sirtuin genes. This is a revolutionary idea that contradicts the prevailing dogma of our time. As part of a healthy diet that tells us to eat two cups of fruit and two and a half cups of vegetables a day, it is time to let go of the generic, blanket guidance. We just have to look around and see how little impact it has had.

Something else became evident with this change in deciding whether plant foods are good for us. In fact, the many foods that supposedly health experts cautioned us about, such as chocolate, coffee, and tea, are so abundant in sirtuin-activating polyphenols that they beat most fruits and vegetables out there. How many times are we grimacing as we swallow our vegetables because we are told that this is the right thing to do, only to feel guilty if we even look at the chocolate treat after dinner? The ultimate irony is that cacao is one of the best foods that we might be eating. Its intake has now been shown to activate sirtuin genes, with several benefits for regulating body weight by burning fat, reducing appetite, and enhancing muscle function. And that's before we take into account its multitude of other health benefits, more of which will come later.

In total, we have identified twenty polyphenol-rich foods that have been shown to activate our sirtuin genes, and together these form the basis of the Sirtfood Diet. While the story began with red wine as the original Sirtfood, for their sirtuin-activating polyphenol content, we now know those other nineteen foods match or trump it. In addition to chocolate, these include other well-known and enjoyable foods such as extra virgin olive oil, red onions, garlic, parsley, chilies, kale, strawberries, walnuts, capers, tofu, green tea, and even coffee. Although food has amazing health credentials of its own, as we are about to see, when we combine these foods to make a whole diet, the real magic happens.

A connection between the healthiest diets in the world

As we further researched, we found that the best sources of sirtfoods were found in the diets of those with the lowest disease and obesity levels in the world — from the Kuna American Indians, who appear immune to high blood pressure and display surprisingly low rates of obesity, diabetes, cancer and early death, thanks to a fantastically rich intake of Sirtfood cocoa; to Okinawa, Japan,

But it is the diet that is the envy of the rest of the Western world, a conventional Mediterranean diet where the benefits of Sirtfoods really stand out. Here, obesity simply does not prevail, and the exception is a chronic disease, not the norm. All-powerful syrups are extra virgin olive oil, wild leafy greens, nuts, berries, red wine, dates, and spices, all featured prominently in Mediterranean native diets. Despite the new consensus that a Mediterranean diet is more effective than calorie counting for weight loss and more effective than prescription medications to avoid disease, the medical community has been left in awe.

This takes us to the 2013 issue of PREDIMED, a Mediterranean Diet game-changing study. It was done on about 7,400 people at high risk of cardiovascular disease, and the findings were so positive that the experiment was eventually stopped early — after only five years. The idea of PREDIMED was gorgeously simple. This questioned what would be the difference between a Mediterranean-style diet supplemented with either extra virgin olive oil or nuts (especially walnuts) and a more traditional modern-day diet. And what sort of a difference. The change in the diet reduced the incidence of cardiovascular disease by around 30 percent, so drug companies can only dream of an outcome. Following further follow-up, there was also a 30 percent drop in diabetes, along with significant drops in inflammation, improvements in memory and brain health, and a massive 40 percent reduction in obesity, with significant fat loss, especially around the stomach area.

But, initially, researchers were unable to explain what such drastic benefits were. Neither the amounts of calories, fats, and sugars consumed — the normal measures used to assess the food we consume — nor the rates of physical activity measured between groups to explain outcomes. There was something else I had to get moving.

Then, eureka moment struck. Both extra virgin olive oil and walnuts are notable for their exceptional polyphenol content, which activates sirtuin. Essentially, by adding these in substantial amounts to a normal Mediterranean diet, what the researchers unwittingly created was a super-rich Sirtfood diet, and they found it delivered incredible results.

The original theory originated from PREDIMED-analyzing researchers. If ultimately it's the polyphenols that count, they mused, then by living the longest, those who eat more of them would gain their accumulated benefits. But the numbers were going, and the results were incredible. Those who drank the highest amounts of polyphenol had 37 percent fewer deaths in just five years than those who ate the lowest. Intriguingly, this is double the reduction in mortality, which is found to bring in treatment with the most commonly prescribed blockbuster statin drugs. Finally, in this study, we had an explanation of the mind-blowing advantages observed, and it was more potent than any existing drug.

The researchers also noticed something else important. While many studies have previously found that individual Sirtfoods confer impressive health benefits, they have never been profound enough to actually extend life. The first such person was PREDIMED. The difference was that they were not looking at a single meal but at a food trend. Different foods have different polyphenols, which cause sirtuin, which functions in conjunction to generate a result that is much more successful than any single food would. It's left us with an irrepressible impression. True health is not caught by a single nutrient or even a "wonder food." What's needed is a complete diet filled with a combination of synergistic Sirtfoods that all work. And this is what contributed to the introduction of the Sirtfood Diet.

The Pilot Study on Sirtfood

Bit by bit, all the results from conventional societies and the findings from major scientific research have been gathered, resulting in PREDIMED, one of the best dietary research studies ever. But even findings from PREDIMED came through chance, just as many health breakthroughs did. It never set out to devise a Sirtfood diet and test it. Science found out much later this that was just what PREDIMED had done. This meant that many Sirtfoods had not been included in the diet, which might have further increased its immense benefits.

Furthermore, all of the research to date has documented the effects of long-term weight loss and disease prevention. But we also did not know how easily such benefits for body weight and health could be realized. In the future we all want to protect our protection but do we not want to look and feel good here and now? To address these questions, we needed an experiment intentionally carried out by the Sirtfood Diet, which included all twenty of the most effective sirtfoods for which we could collect measurements of earlier tests. And we started our own pilot test.

Nestled in the south of London, England, KX is one of Europe's most sought-after recreation and fitness centers. That makes K.X. The perfect place to test the effects of the Sirtfood Diet is that it has its own restaurant, which has given us the opportunity not only to design the diet but also to bring it to life and test it on the fitness center members. Our know-how was clear. Members would follow our carefully designed Sirtfood Diet for seven days in a row, and we would closely monitor their progress from beginning to end, not only measuring their weight but also tracking changes in their body composition, including testing how the diet influenced the body's fat and muscle levels. Later on, we added metabolic measures to see the effects of the diet on blood sugar (glucose) levels and fats (such as triglycerides and cholesterol).

The first three days were the most intense, with a food intake limited to one thousand calories a day. Because the lower energy intake slows down signals of growth in the body and allows it to start clearing out old debris from cells (a process known as autophagy) and kick-starting fat burning, yet this fast was mild and short-lived, unlike conventional fasting diets, making it much more manageable, as seen by the remarkably high adherence rate of 97.5 percent of the study. Furthermore, we have decided to explore the variations created by introducing Sirtfoods into the common falls associated with fasting diets. And they were dramatic, as we were to find out very soon.

Our primary goal was to make a major difference to the fat-burning effects of this moderate calorie restriction by packing a diet full of Sirtfood. This was achieved by basing the daily diet on three Sirtfood-rich green drinks, and one Sirtfood-rich meal.

At K.X. for the last four days of our program, calories were raised to 1,500 per day. This was, in fact, only a very mild calorie deficit, but it turned down, and fat-burning signals turned up enough to keep signals of growth. Importantly, Sirtfoods had a jam-packed 1,500-calorie diet, consisting of two Sirtfood-rich green juices and two Sirtfood-rich meals a day.

The Amazing Results

The Sirtfood Diet was checked at K.X. By 40 people and completed by 39 participants. Of these 39, two were obese in the trial, fifteen were overweight, and twenty-two had a normal/healthy body mass index (BMI). The sample was divided relatively even in gender, with twenty-one women and eighteen men. Being members of a health club, they were more likely than the general population to exercise and be aware of healthy eating before they started. A trick of many diets is to use a heavily overweight and unhealthy sample of people to show the benefits, because at first, they lose weight the fastest and most dramatically, essentially fluffing up the diet results. Our reasoning was the opposite: if we obtained successful results with this fairly safe community, the minimum benchmark of what was achievable would be set.

The results far exceeded our expectations, which were already high. The results were consistent and astonishing: an average weight loss of 7 pounds in seven days following muscle gain accounting. As if that wasn't admirable enough, we've seen something else even more impressive, which was the weight loss type. Usually, when people lose weight, they're going to lose some fat, but they're going to also lose some muscle — this is par for the diet course. We were amazed to discover the opposite. Our participants either kept their muscles or gained muscle. This is an even more desirable form of weight loss, and a special feature of the Sirtfood Diet, as we will find out later in the book.

No individual struggled to see body structure changes. And note, without dietary deprivation or grueling workout regimens, all this was accomplished.

Here's what we got:
- Dramatic and quick results were achieved by the participants, losing an average of 7 pounds in seven days.
- Weight loss around the abdominal area was most noticeable.
- The muscle mass was either maintained or increased; it was not lost.
- Rarely did the participants feel hungry.
- Participants felt a stronger sense of health and wellness.
- Participants reported a healthier look and look better.

Diet in the Real World

It is one thing to get great results after a diet in a controlled environment where all the food is made and delivered expertly, and nutrition experts are on hand to answer any queries. When people are left to fend for themselves with nothing more to help them, it's something else altogether that can be found on the pages of this very book. But those reports were the ones that really blew our minds — a diet that can so effectively encourage weight loss and boost body structure; it also has many useful applications for turbocharging energy levels and health. Hundreds of testimonials had sprinkled in before long. From sports superstars who were world champions and Olympic gold medalists to television celebrities and models to showbiz's biggest names, they not only embraced it and stuck to it, but they were raving about it.

Readers smashed the 7 pounds we'd seen in our trial in seven days of weight loss, proving our hypothesis that our already-fit and healthy study population underestimated the benefits. The maximum weight loss we have seen so far was with a reporter and diet cynic, who set out to test the merits of the program independently. He lost 14 pounds in the first week, instead of bad-mouthing it, he was fair enough to assume that he now joins the convert cohorts. Others reported equally impressive results, away from the scales, by inches lost around the waist. And best of all, the weight stayed off, with results only improving over the months.

As fantastic as all this feedback was, there was something that inspired us even more for us as nutritional medicine consultants who specialize in reversing and preventing disease: the personal stories that, just like Racheal's at the beginning of this chapter, was nothing short of life-changing.

There was Greg, who'd suffered for years from depression. In only two weeks, he lost 10 pounds but was much more pleased with the lifting of his depressed mood, so much so that he was once again "doing life." Melanie was suffering terrible lupus pain. She was down 11.5 pounds five weeks later, but even more importantly, her pains and aches had vanished. Indeed she had no symptoms of lupus at all. She felt great and didn't have to go to her doctor anymore; there was nothing to treat. And Linda, who after three months had been down an astounding 50 pounds, reversed her deteriorating diabetes and had the ability to enjoy life once again. That's just a taste of the many inspiring stories that's come in. Heart disease has gone backward. Symptoms of menopause have ceased. Irritable conditions in the bowel have gone missing. People were sleeping fine again for the first time in years. One perplexed ophthalmologist also approached us with the news that the chronic discoloration of her patient's sclera had absolutely reversed after only a week on the Sirtfood Diet and was now fully white again. She also sent photos to prove it.

How The Sirtfood Diet Will Work For You

The sheer breadth of benefits experienced by people has been a revelation, all achieved by simply basing their diet on accessible and affordable foods that most people already enjoy eating. And that is all that the Sirtfood Diet needs. It's about extracting the benefits of daily foods that we've all been meant to consume, but in the right amounts and combinations to give us the body structure and well-being that we all desire so desperately, and that can eventually improve our lives. It doesn't require you to execute severe calorie restrictions, nor does it require grueling exercise regimens (although generally staying active is a good thing, of course). And just a juicer is the only piece of equipment you'll need. Plus, unlike any other diet out there that focuses on what to exclude, the Sirtfood Diet focuses on what to include.

The Sirtfood Diet will help you to sum up all this:
- Lose weight, not muscle, by burning fat
- Burning fat, particularly from the stomach, to feel healthier
- Prime your body to long-term success in weight loss
- See and look stronger, and get more strength
- Do not endure severe calorie or extreme hunger
- Be free from cumbersome exercise regimes
- Living a longer, healthier and sicker life

CHAPTER ONE: SIRTUINS STUDIES

What makes the Sirtfood Diet so powerful is its ability to switch to an ancient gene family that exists within each of us. The name for that gene family is sirtuin. Sirtuins are unique because they orchestrate processes deep within our cells that affect such important things as our ability to burn fat, our vulnerability to disease — or not — and ultimately, even our life span. The effect of sirtuins is so profound that they are now referred to as "master metabolic regulators. "1 In essence, what exactly anyone who wants to shed some pounds and live a long and healthy life would want to be in charge of.

Of Mice and Men

In recent years, sirtuins have, understandably, become the subject of intense scientific research. The first sirtuin was discovered in yeast back in 1984, and research really began over the next three decades when it was revealed that sirtuin activation improves life span, first in yeast, and then all the way up to mice. Why the thrills? It is because the basic principles of cellular metabolism are almost identical from mice to humans, and everything in between. If you can manipulate something as tiny as budding yeast and see a benefit, then repeat it in higher organisms like mice, there is potential for the same benefits to be realized in humans.

Sirtfood and an Appetite for Fasting

That leads us to speed. It has been shown repeatedly that the lifelong restriction of food consumption increases the life span of lower organisms and mammals; This remarkable finding for certain people is the basis of the practice of caloric restriction, where daily calorie intake is reduced by around 20 to 30%, as well as its popularized offshoot, intermittent fasting, which has become an effective weight-loss diet. While we are still waiting for evidence from these practices of increased lifespan for humans, there is evidence of benefits to what we might call "healthspan"— chronic disease drops, and fat begins to melt away.

But let's be honest, no matter how huge the rewards, it's a grueling company that most of us don't want to sign up for, fasting week in, week out. Even though we do, most of us can not stick to this. Besides this, fasting has its disadvantages, especially if we follow it for a long time to come. In the introduction, we described the side effects of hunger, irritability, tiredness, muscle loss, and metabolism slowdown. Nevertheless, ongoing fasting schemes may also put us at risk of malnutrition, affecting our well-being as a result of reduced vital nutrient intakes. Fasting schemes are also totally inadequate for large proportions of the population, such as children, women during pregnancy, and very possibly the elderly. While fasting has clearly demonstrated benefits, it isn't the magic bullet we would like it to be. It had us ask, was this really the way nature was supposed to make us safe and thin? Sure there's a better way out there.

Our discovery came when we discovered that the profound benefits of caloric restriction and fasting were mediated by triggering our ancient sirtuin genes.5 To better understand this, it may be beneficial to think of the sirtuins as the guardians at the crossroads of energy status and longevity. There, what they are doing is responding to stress, that is, when energy is in short supply, the stress on our cells increases exactly as we see in the calorie constraint. This was sensed by the sirtuins, which then turned on and transmitted a series of powerful signals that dramatically altered cell behavior. Sirtuins ramp up our metabolism, increase our muscle capacity, turn on fat burning, decrease inflammation, and repair any cell damage. In turn, the sirtuins make us fitter, leaner, and healthier.

Seven distinct sirtuins (SIRT1 to SIRT7) exist in humans. For these, SIRT1 and SIRT3 are the two main sirtuins involved in energy balance. Although SIRT1 is present throughout the body, SIRT3 is found mainly in the energy-powerhouses of our mitochondria — the cells. Their joint activation gives us the many benefits we are looking to achieve.

Do You Have a Passion for Exercise?

It's not just caloric restriction and fasting that activates sirtuins; exercise does too.6 Sirtuins orchestrate the profound benefits of exercise, just as they do in fasting. But while we are encouraged to engage in regular, moderate exercise for its multitude of benefits, it is not the means by which we are intended to focus our efforts on weight-loss.

Research shows that the human body has evolved ways of adjusting naturally and reducing the amount of energy that we expend when exercising, seven meaning that for exercise to be an effective weight-loss intervention, we need to commit considerable time and effort. Those grueling exercise regimens are the way nature intended us to maintain a healthy weight is even more dubious in the light of research now suggesting that exercising too much can be harmful — weakening our immune systems, harming the heart, and contributing to an early death.

Diving Into Sirtfood

So far, we have found that if we want to lose weight and be healthy, the key to activating our sirtuin genes is to eat diets that activate these genes. Until now, fasting and exercise were the two known ways to do this. Unfortunately, the sums required for a good weight loss come with their disadvantages, and for most of us, this is simply inconsistent with how we live lives in the 21st century. Fortunately, there's a groundbreaking newly discovered way to activate our sirtuin genes in the best possible way: sirtfood. As we will soon know, these are the wonder foods that are especially rich in unique natural plant chemicals, which have the power to talk to and turn on our sirtuin genes. By turn, they imitate the previously unattainable effects of fasting and exercise and, in so doing, offer incredible benefits of burning fat, building muscles, and health-boosting.

Let's Wrap This Up!
- We each have an ancient family of genes named sirtuins.
- Master metabolic regulators are sirtuins that regulate our fat-burning capacity and remain healthy.
- Sirtuins serve as energy sensors in our cells and enable the detection of energy shortages.
- Fasting and exercise both activate our sirtuin genes, but may be hard to adhere to, and may even have disadvantages.
- In a new revolutionary way, our sirtuin genes are activated: sirtfoods.
- You can mimic the effects of fasting and exercise by eating a Sirtfood rich diet and achieving the body you want.

CHAPTER TWO: FIGHTING FAT

One of the dramatic findings from our Sirtfood Diet pilot study wasn't just how much weight the participants lost, which was impressive enough — it was the type of weight loss that really excited us. What caught our attention was the fact that a lot of people lost weight without losing any muscle. In fact, seeing people gain muscle wasn't uncommon. This left us with an unavoidable conclusion: fat had merely melted away.

Achieving a significant fat loss normally requires a considerable sacrifice, either severely reducing calories or engaging in superhuman exercise levels, or both. But contrary to that, our participants either maintained or lowered their level of exercise and did not even report feeling especially hungry. In fact, some even struggled to eat all of the food they had been provided with. How is it even that possible? It is only when we understand what happens to our fat cells when there is increased sirtuin activity that we can begin to make sense of these remarkable results.

The Lean Genes

Mice that have been genetically engineered to have high SIRT1 levels are leaner and more metabolically active, the sirtuin gene that causes fat loss, whereas mice that lack SIRT1 are fatter and have more metabolic disease. When we look at humans, levels of SIRT1 in obese people's body fat have been found to be considerably lower compared to their healthy-weight counterparts. In contrast, lower levels of SIRT1 have been found in humans.

Stack all that up, and you start to get a sense of just how important sirtuins are to decide whether we stay lean or get fat and why through sirtuin activity, you can produce such impressive results. This is because, through sirtuins, we get advantages on several levels, beginning at the very root of everything: the genes that obtain weight regulation. To fully understand this, we need to look deeper into what's going on in our bodies, which is causing us to gain some weight.

Busting Fat

We'll explain this in terms of a drug-ring film in Hollywood. The streets flooding with drugs is our body flooding with fat. The drug pushers on the street corners are the source of the weight gain peddling reactions in our bodies. But in reality, it's just the low-level thugs. The true villain is behind it all, masterminding the entire operation, directing every deal that the peddlers make. This villain is referred to in our film as PPAR-π (peroxisome proliferator-activated receptor-ÿ). PPAR-ÿ orchestrates the cycle of fat production by switching on the genes needed to start synthesizing and storing fat. To avoid fat proliferation, you need to cut supply. Stop PPAR-ÿ, and you avoid fat build-up effectively.

Enter our hero SIRT1, who rises to put the villain down. With the villain locked up safely, there's no one to pull the trigger, and the whole fat-gain enterprise crumbles. With PPAR-π's operation halted, SIRT1 shifts its focus to "cleaning the streets." Not only is this achieved by shutting down fat output and storage, as we have shown, but it also alters our metabolism so that we begin to clear the body of excess fat. Like any good crime-fighting hero, SIRT1 has a sidekick, a central regulator in our cells named PGC-1α. This powerfully stimulates the establishment of what is known as mitochondria. They are the tiny factories of energy that exist within each of our cells — they power the body. The more we have the mitochondria, the more we can produce the energy. But as well as promoting more mitochondria, PGC-1α also encourages them to burn fat as the fuel of choice to make the energy. Thus fat storage is blocked on the one hand, and fat burning on the other increases.

BAT or WAT?

We have looked so far at the effects of SIRT1 on fat loss on a well-known fat type called white adipose tissue (WAT). This is the type of fat that weight gain associates with. It specializes in storage and expansion, is horribly stubborn, and secretes a host of inflammatory chemicals that resist fat burning and stimulate the further accumulation of fat, making us overweight and obese. That's why weight gain often starts slowly but is able to snowball so fast.

But the sirtuin story has another intriguing angle, involving a lesser-known type of fat, brown adipose tissue (BAT), which behaves quite differently. BAT is beneficial to us in complete contrast to white adipose tissue and wants to get used up. Brown adipose tissue actually helps us expend energy and has developed into mammals to allow them to dissipate large quantities of heat-shaped fat. This is known as a thermogenic influence and is important to help small mammals survive in cold temperatures. Babies also possess considerable amounts of brown adipose tissue in humans, although it decreases shortly after birth, leaving smaller amounts in adults.

This is where the activation of SIRT1 is doing something truly amazing. It changes genes in our white adipose tissue to transform and adapt the properties of brown adipose tissue in what is called a "browning effect." This means that our fat stores begin to act in a radically different way — instead of storing energy, they start mobilizing it to be disposed of.

Sirtuin activation, as we can see, has a potent direct action on fat cells, encouraging the fat to melt away. But there, it's not over. The sirtuins also have a beneficial effect on the most important weight reduction hormones. Sirtuin activation improves insulin activity. This helps reduce insulin resistance — the inability of our cells to respond to insulin properly — which is heavily implicated in weight gain. SIRT1 also enhances our thyroid hormones' release and activity, which share many overlapping roles in boosting our metabolism and, ultimately, the rate at which we burn fat.

Controlling Your Appetite

There was one thing we couldn't wrap our heads around in our pilot study: the participants didn't really get hungry despite a reduction in calories. In fact, some people struggled to eat all of the food that was provided. One of the major advantages of the Sirtfood Diet is that without the need for a long-term calorie restriction, we can reap great benefits. The very first week of diet is the phase of hyper-success, where we combine moderate fasting with an abundance of powerful Sirtfoods for a double blow to fat. And we expected some signs of hunger here, as with all of the fasting regimens. But we've had absolutely none!

We found the answer, as we trawled through analysis. It's all thanks to the body's main appetite-regulating hormone, leptin, called the "satiety hormone." As we feed, leptin rises, signaling the hypothalamus inhibiting desire to a section of the brain. Conversely, leptin signaling to the brain decreases when we fly, and this makes us feel hungry.

Leptin is so effective in controlling appetite that early expectations were it could be used as a "magic bullet" for treating obesity. But that dream was shattered by the realization that the metabolic dysfunction occurring in obesity actually causes leptin to stop properly working. Through obesity, the amount of leptin that can enter the brain is not only decreased, but the hypothalamus often becomes desensitized to its behavior. This is known as leptin resistance: there is leptin, but it doesn't work properly anymore. Thus, for many overweight individuals, the brain continues to think they are underfed even though they eat enough, and signals for them to continue to seek food.

The consequence of this is that while the amount of leptin in the blood is necessary to control appetite, how much of it enters the brain and can have an effect on the hypothalamus is much more relevant. It is here that the Sirtfoods shine. Recent research suggests that the nutrients present in Sirtfoods have specific advantages in reversing leptin resistance. This is by both increasing leptin delivery to the brain and improving the hypothalamus' responsiveness to leptin behavior. So back to our original question: Why doesn't the Sirtfood Diet make people feel hungry? Given a drop in blood leptin levels during the mild quick, which would usually increase hunger, incorporating Sirtfoods into the diet makes leptin signals more effective, leading to better control of appetite.

As we'll see later, Sirtfoods also have powerful effects on our taste centers, meaning we get a lot more pleasure and satisfaction from our food and therefore don't fall into the overeating trap to feel happy.

Sirtuin is likely to be a brand-new concept for even the most dedicated dietitians. But targeting the sirtuins, our metabolism's master regulators, is the cornerstone of any effective weight-loss diet. Tragically, the very nature of our modern society, with abundant food and sedentary lifestyles, creates a perfect storm to shut down our sirtuin activity, and we see all around us the consequences of this. The good news is that we now know what sirtuins are, how fat storage is managed, and how fat burning is encouraged, and, most importantly, how to turn them on. And with this groundbreaking breakthrough, the key to successful and enduring weight loss is finally yours to take.

- Let's Wrap This Up!
- Fat on a Sirtfood Diet melts away. This is because sirtuins have the power to determine if we remain lean or are getting fat.

- SIRT1 activation inhibits PPAR-ÿ, blocking fat production and storage.
- SIRT1 activation also turns on PGC-1α, which makes our cells more power plants and increases fat burning.
- Activating SIRT1 even results in our fat cells, which are specialized in energy storage, behaving differently, and starting energy disposal.
- Sirtfood diet is unlikely to make you feel hungry because it helps to regulate your brain's appetite.

CHAPTER THREE: THE WONDERS OF WELL-BEING

Despite all the amazing advances in modern medicine, society is getting fatter and sicker—70 percent of all deaths are due to chronic disease, truly shocking statistics. Change is required radically and rapidly. Yet as we have seen, this can all start to change. By activating our old sirtuin genes, we can burn fat and develop a leaner, stronger body. And with sirtuins at the center of our metabolism, our master programmers in biology, their importance reaches well beyond the structure of the body alone, to every dimension of our health.

Sirtuins and the 70 percent remaining

Think of a disease that you associate with getting old, and the chances are that the body lacks sirtuin activity. For example, sirtuin activation is great for cardiac health, protecting the muscle cells in the heart, and generally improving the functioning of the heart muscle. It also enhances how our arteries operate, enables us to manage cholesterol more effectively, and protects our arteries, known as atherosclerosis, against blockage.

Diabetes as it were? Activation of the sirtuin increases the amount of insulin that can be secreted and helps it to act more efficiently within the body. As it happens, one of the most popular antidiabetic drugs, metformin, relies on SIRT1 for its beneficial effect. Yes, one pharmaceutical company is currently investigating the application of natural sirtuin activators to diabetic metformin care, with findings from animal trials showing a staggering 83 percent reduction in the dose of metformin needed for the same effects.

As for the brain, sirtuins are involved once again, with sirtuin activity found to be lower in Alzheimer's patients. By contrast, sirtuin activation enhances communication signals within the brain, enhances cognitive function, and reduces brain inflammation. This prevents the accumulation of amyloid-β development and the aggregation of tau proteins, two of the most damaging things we see happening in the brains of Alzheimer's patients.

Such are the bones. Osteoblasts are a special type of cell that is responsible for forming new bone in our bodies. The more we acquire osteoblasts, the stronger our bones are. Sirtuin activation not only promotes osteoblast cell production but also increases its survival. That makes sirtuin activation essential to lifelong bone health.

Cancer has been a more controversial area for sirtuin research, and while recent research shows that sirtuin activation helps to suppress cancer tumors, scientists are only beginning to unravel this complex field. While there is much more to learn about this particular topic, those crops that eat most Sirtfoods have the lowest cancer rates, as we will see soon. Heart disease, diabetes, arthritis, osteoporosis, and cancer most likely make up a fascinating list of diseases that sirtuin activation can avoid. It may come as no surprise to find out that communities that already consume plenty of Sirtfood as part of their conventional diets are experiencing resilience and well-being that most of us can hardly imagine, which you will hear more about very soon.

That leaves us with an exciting conclusion: simply by adding to your diet the best sirt foods in the world and making it a lifelong habit, you too can experience this degree of well-being — and more — while having the physics you want.

Let's Wrap This Up!
- Despite all the advances in modern medicine, we are getting fatter and sicker as a society.
- Chronic illness accounts for 70 % of all deaths, with low sirtuin activity involved in the vast majority.
- You can prevent or forestall major Western chronic diseases by activating sirtuins.
- You, too, will achieve the same degree of well-being as the healthiest and longest-living communities on the planet by loading your diet full of Sirtfoods.

CHAPTER FOUR: TYPES OF SIRTFOODS

We've discovered so far that sirtuins are an ancient gene family with the power to help us burn fat, build muscle, and keep us super-healthy. It is well known that through caloric restriction, fasting, and exercise, sirtuins can be turned on, but there is another innovative way to accomplish this: food. We refer to the most potent foods to activate sirtuins as Sirtfoods.

Beyond Antioxidants

To really understand the benefits of Sirtfoods, we need to think about foods like fruits and vegetables very differently, and why they are good for us. Despite tons of evidence testifying that diets high in fruits, vegetables, and processed products usually cut the risk of many chronic diseases, including the biggest killers, heart disease, and cancer, there is absolutely no denying they do. It has been put down to their rich nutritional content, such as vitamins, minerals, and, of course, antioxidants, which is perhaps the biggest wellness buzzword of the last decade. But this is a very different story we are here to tell.

The reason Sirtfoods is so good for you has nothing to do with the nutrients that we all know so well and hear about so much. Yes, they're all important items you need to get out of your diet, but with Sirtfoods, there's something completely different and very unique. In fact, what if we threw that whole way of thinking on its head and said that the reason Sirtfoods is good for you is not that they nourish the body with essential nutrients, or provide antioxidants to mop up the damaging effects of free radicals, but quite the opposite: because they are full of weak toxins? It could sound insane in a world where almost every alleged "superfood" is actively promoted based on its antioxidant content. Yet it's a novel concept, and one worth taking on.

What Does Not Kill You Makes You Stronger

Let's get back to the known manner of triggering sirtuins for a moment: fasting and exercise. Research has shown repeatedly, as we have shown, that dietary energy restriction has significant benefits for weight loss, health, and, quite likely, longevity. There is also exercise, with its various advantages for both body and mind, borne out by the discovery that routine exercise significantly slashes mortality rates. So what are they all sharing in common?

The answer is Stress. All that fasting and exercise create is a slight stress on the body, which helps the body to adapt by being fitter, more productive, and more resilient. It is the body's response to these mildly stressful stimuli — their adaptation — that makes us fitter, healthier, and leaner in the long run. And as we now know, sirtuins orchestrate these highly beneficial adaptations that are turned on in the face of those stressors and spark a host of desirable body changes.

The scientific term used to respond to such stresses is hormesis. It's the idea that if exposed to a low dose of a substance or stress that is otherwise toxic or lethal if given at higher doses, you get a beneficial effect. Or "what doesn't kill you makes you stronger," if you prefer. And that's exactly how fasting and exercise work. Hunger is lethal, and excessive exercise is prejudicial to health. These extreme forms of stress are clearly harmful, but they have highly beneficial effects as long as fasting and exercise remain moderate and manageable tresses.

Polyphenols

Now, here's where things really get interesting. All living organisms undergo hormesis, but what has been significantly underestimated until now is that it also involves plants. While we may not usually think of plants as being the same as other living organisms, let alone humans, we do share similar responses in terms of how we respond to our environment on a chemical level.

As mind-blowing as that sounds, it makes complete sense to think evolutionarily about it, as all living organisms have evolved to encounter and cope with common environmental stresses such as starvation, heat, lack of nutrients, and pathogens assault. If that's hard to wrap your head around, get ready for the truly incredible part. Plant stress responses are more complex indeed than ours. Think about it: if we're hungry and thirsty, we can go in search of food and drink; too dry, we'll need shade; under attack, we can run. In absolute comparison, plants are stationary, and as such, must tolerate all the severity of these physiological stresses and challenges. As a result, over the past billion years, they have developed a highly sophisticated stress-response system that humbles everything we can boast about. The way they do this is to produce a vast collection of natural plant chemicals — called polyphenols — that will enable them to adapt and survive successfully in their environment. When we eat these plants, we also consume those polyphenol nutrients. Their effect is profound: To respond to stress, they activate our own innate pathways. This is precisely the same paths that turn on to fasting and exercise: the sirtuins.

To our own benefit, piggybacking on a plant's stress-response system is thus known as xenohormesis. And the implications of that are changing the game. Let the plants do the hard work, and we don't need to. Indeed, because of their ability to turn on the same positive changes in our cells, such as fat burning, which would be seen during fasting, these natural plant compounds are now referred to as caloric restriction mimetics. And by supplying us with more sophisticated signaling compounds than we actually produce, they cause results that are superior to anything we can accomplish by fasting or exercising on our own.

Foods that are grown in the wild, or even organically, are better for us than intensively farmed produce because they produce higher levels of polyphenols because of a greater need to adapt to survive in their environment.

Sirtfoods

Although all plants have these stress-response systems, only some have evolved to produce remarkable amounts of sirtuin-activating polyphenols. We call some plants, Sirtfoods. Their discovery means that now there is a groundbreaking new way to trigger the sirtuin genes in place of austere fasting regimes or arduous workout programs: consuming an ample diet in Sirtfoods. Best of all, this one involves putting on your plate (Sirt)food, not removing it!

It's so beautifully simple, and it looks so easy it needs a catch. But this is not so. This is how nature intended us to eat, rather than the rumbling count of modern diet in the stomach or calories. Many of you who have experienced those hellish diets, where the initial weight loss is fleeting before the body rebels and the weight piles up again, will understandably shudder at the thought of another false promise, another book boasting the dreaded "d" word. But remember this: the modern dietary approach is only 150 years old; Nature developed Sirtfoods more than a billion years ago.

And you are probably itching with that to know what Sirtfoods counts for specific foods. So, here's the top twenty Sirtfoods with no more ado.

Let's wrap this up!
- We must fundamentally reconsider the notion that fruits, vegetables, and plant products are healthy for us simply because they contain vitamins and antioxidants;
- They're good for us because they contain natural chemicals that put a little stress on our cells, just like fasting and exercise.
- Plants have built a highly sophisticated stress-response mechanism as they are stationary, generating polyphenols to help them respond to their environment's challenges.
- When we eat these plants, their polyphenols activate our stress-response pathways — our sirtuin genes — to mimic and exert the effects of caloric restraint.
- Sirtfoods are the most potent sirtuin-activating foods.

CHAPTER FIVE: BUILDING A HEALTHY DIET THAT WORKS

We are doing something very special with the Sirtfood Diet. We took the most powerful Sirtfoods on the planet and woven them into a brand-new way of eating, the likes of which were never seen before. We picked the "best of the best" from the healthiest diets we have ever seen and built a world-beating diet from them. The good news is, you don't immediately have to follow an Okinawan's typical diet or cook like an Italian mamma. That on the Sirtfood Diet is not only utterly unrealistic but totally unnecessary. Indeed, one thing you may be struck by from the Sirtfoods list is their familiarity. While you might not consume any of the foods on the list at the moment, you are most likely eating some. So why don't you just lose weight already?

The response is found when we explore the various elements that the most cutting-edge nutrition science shows are required to create a workable diet. It is about eating the right amount of Sirtfoods, variety, and shape. It's about adding generous protein servings to the Sirtfood dishes and then eating your meals at the best time of day. And it's about the freedom to eat the genuinely savory foods you enjoy in the quantities you like.

Hit Your Quota

Most people just don't consume nearly enough Sirtfoods right now to elicit a potent fat-burning and health-boosting effect. When researchers looked at the intake of five key sirtuin-activating nutrients (quercetin, myricetin, kaempferol, luteolin, and apigenin) in the U.S. diet, they found individual daily intakes to be miserably 13 milligrams per day.1 In contrast, Japan's average intake was five times higher.2 Compare that with our Sirtfood Diet trial, where people consumed hundreds of milligrams of sirtuin-activating nutrients daily.

What we are talking about is a total diet revolution in which we increase by as much as fifty times our daily intake of sirtuin-activating nutrients. While that may sound daunting or impractical, it isn't really. By taking all our top Sirtfoods and bringing them together in a way that is completely consistent with your busy life, you too can easily and effectively achieve the amount of intake needed to reap all of the benefits.

The Power of Synergy

We believe it is best to eat a wide variety of these wonderful nutrients as whole natural foods, where they coexist alongside the hundreds of other natural bioactive plant chemicals that work synergistically to improve our well-being. We think working with nature is better, rather than against it. It is for this reason that isolated nutrient supplements do not show lasting benefit time and time again, yet the same nutrient is provided in the form of an entire food.

Take, for example, the classic nutrient resveratrol, which activates sirtuin. In addition, it is poorly absorbed; but its bioavailability (how much the body can use) is at least six times higher in its natural food matrix of red wine. Add to this the fact that red wine contains not just one but a whole range of sirtuin-activating polyphenols that combine to bring health benefits, including piceatannol, quercetin, myricetin, and epicatechin. Or we could turn our attention from the turmeric to curcumin. Curcumin is well-established as the key sirtuin-activating nutrient in turmeric, but research shows that whole turmeric has better fat loss control activity and is more effective in inhibiting cancer and lowering blood sugar levels than isolated curcumin. It is not difficult to see why isolating a single nutrient is nowhere near as efficient as consuming it in its entire diet.

But what really makes a dietary approach different is when we start mixing multiple Sirtfoods. For example, we further enhance the bioavailability of resveratrol-containing foods by adding them to quercetin-rich Sirtfoods. Not only this, but they complement each other with their actions. All are fat busters, but there are variations of how every one of them is doing this. Resveratrol is very effective in helping to kill existing fat cells, while quercetin excels in preventing the development of new fat cells.6 In addition, both sides target fat, resulting in a greater impact on the loss of fat than only consuming large amounts of a single food.

And this is a pattern that we see again and again. Foods rich in sirtuin activator *apigenin* increase the absorption of quercetin from food and enhance its activity. In addition, quercetin has been shown to synergize with epigallocatechin gallate (EGCG) activity. And it has been shown that EGCG acts synergistically with curcumin. And so it continues. Not only are individual whole foods more powerful than isolated nutrients, but we tap into a whole tapestry of health benefits that nature has weaved — so complex, so refined, it's impossible to try to trump it.

Food and Juicing: Get the best of both worlds

Sirtfood Diet is a component of both juices and whole foods. We're thinking here about juices made directly from a juicer — blenders and smoothie makers (such as the NutriBullet) won't function. For many, this will seem counterintuitive, based on the fact that the fiber is removed when something is juiced. But this is exactly what we want for leafy greens. Food fiber contains what is termed non-extractable polyphenols (or NEPPs). There are polyphenols, called sirtuin activators, which are bound to the fibrous portion of the food and only released by our friendly gut bacteria when broken down. We don't get the NEPPs by removing the fiber and lose out on their goodness. Importantly, however, the NEPP content varies dramatically depending on the plant type. The NEPP content of foods such as fruit, cereals, and nuts is significant and should be eaten whole (NEPPs provide over 50 percent of polyphenols in strawberries!). But for leafy vegetables, the active ingredients in the Sirtfood juice are much lower despite having high fiber content.

So when it comes to leafy greens, by juicing them and removing the low-nutrient fiber, we get maximum bang for our buck, meaning we can use much larger volumes and achieve a superconcentrated hit of sirtuin-activating polyphenols. There's another advantage in cutting the thread, too. Leafy greens contain a type of fiber called insoluble fiber, which has a digestive scrubbing action. But when we eat too much of it, it can irritate and hurt our gut lining just as if we over scrub something. That means that for many people, leafy green-packed smoothies will overload fiber, potentially aggravating or even causing IBS (irritable bowel syndrome) and hampering our nutrient absorption.

When it comes to absorbing their goodness, having some of your Sirtfoods in juice form can also have big advantages. For instance, matcha green tea is one of the ingredients we include in the green juice. When we ingest the sirtuin activator EGCG, found at high levels in green tea, in drinking form without food, its absorption is higher than 65 percent.10 We also find it interesting to note that when we performed blood tests on our own clients, switching from smoothies to green juices triggered dramatic increases in their levels of other essential nutrients such as magnesium and folic acid. The crux of it all is that we need to build a diet that combines both juices and whole foods for maximum benefit to really get those sirtuin genes firing for dramatic weight loss and health.

The Might of Protein

It's plants that put the Sirt into the Sirtfood Diet, but Sirtfood meals should always be rich in protein to reap maximum benefit. A dietary protein building block called leucine has been shown to have additional benefits in stimulating SIRT1 to increase fat burning and improve the regulation of blood sugar.

But leucine also has another role, and this is where it really shines through its synergistic relationship with Sirtfoods. Leucine powerfully stimulates anabolism (building things) in our cells, especially in the muscle, which demands a great deal of energy and means that our energy factories (called mitochondria) have to work overtime. This generates a need for the Sirtfoods operation within our cells. As you may recall, one of the effects of Sirtfoods is to stimulate the production of more mitochondria, to improve their efficiency, and to make them burn fat as fuel. Our bodies, therefore, need these to satisfy this extra demand for energy. The upshot is that by combining Sirtfoods with dietary protein, we see a synergistic effect that will boost sirtuin activation and ultimately get you to burn fat to fuel muscle growth and better health. That's why the meals in the book are designed to provide a generous protein serving.

Oily fish is an exceptionally good protein choice to complement Sirtfoods' action because they are rich in omega-3 fatty acids besides their protein content. There is no doubt that you will have heard a lot about the health benefits of oily fish and specifically omega-3 fish oils. And now recent research suggests that the benefits of omega-3 fats can come from improving the way our sirtuin genes work.

In recent years, concerns have been raised about the negative effects of protein-rich diets on health, and without Sirtfoods to counterbalance the protein, we can start to understand why. Leucine may be a knife with two edges. We need Sirtfoods, as we have seen, to help our cells meet the metabolic demand that leucine places upon them.

Without them, however, our mitochondria can become dysfunctional, and high levels of leucine can actually promote obesity and insulin resistance, rather than improve health. Sirtfoods help not only keep the effects of leucine in check but also work effectively in our favor. Think of leucine as pressing your foot on the weight loss and well-being accelerator, with Sirtfoods the machine that ensures that the cell meets the increased demand. The engine blows, without the Sirtfoods.

Returning to concerns over the health effects of protein-rich diets, the missing piece of the puzzle is Sirtfoods. Typically, the U.S. diet is protein-rich but lacks Sirtfoods to counterbalance it. That makes it important for Sirtfoods to become an integral part of how Americans eat.

Eating Early

Our theory is the sooner, the better when it comes to food, preferably done food for the day by 7 p.m. That is on two grounds. Firstly, to reap the Sirtfoods natural satiating effect. Eating a meal that will keep you feeling full, satisfied, and energized as you go about your day is much more beneficial than spending the entire day feeling hungry just to eat and stay full as you sleep through the night.

But there's a second compelling reason to keep eating habits in keeping with your inner body clock. We all have an integrated body clock, called our circadian rhythm, which regulates many of our natural body functions according to daytime. It influences, among other things, how the body handles the food that we eat. Our clocks operate in synchrony, observing mainly the sun's light-dark cycle signals. We're programmed as a diurnal species to be active in the daytime rather than at night. Our body clock, therefore, allows us to manage food more effectively throughout the day when there is light, and we're supposed to be busy, and less so when it's dark when we're prepared for rest and sleep instead.

The problem is that many of us have "work clocks" and "social clocks," which are not synchronized with the sun's powering. Sometimes after dark is the only chance some of us get to eat. To some degree, we can train our body clock to synchronize with various routines like "evening chronotypes" that prefer or need to be involved, eat, and sleep later in the day. Living misaligned from the light-dark external cycle, however, comes at a cost. Studies reveal that individuals with evening chronotype have increased susceptibility to fat gain, muscle loss, and metabolic problems, as well as often suffering from poor sleep. This is exactly what we see among night-shift workers, who have higher rates of obesity and metabolic disease, at least in part due to the effects of their patterns of late eating.

The upshot is that when possible, you're better off eating earlier in the day, ideally by 7 p.m. But what if that is simply not feasible? The good news is that sirtuins play a key part in synchronizing the body clock. In addition, research has found that the polyphenols in Sirtfoods can modulate our body clocks and change circadian rhythm positively. This means that if you actually cannot stop eating later, the inclusion of Sirtfoods with your meal can reduce the adverse effects. Indeed, one of the frequent feedback we hear from Sirtfood Diet followers is just how much their quality of sleep has improved, indicating potent effects on their circadian rhythm harmonization.

Go High On Your Taste

A fundamental problem with a conventional diet is that it typically makes the dining experience miserable. It steals the last drop of food satisfaction and leaves us feeling sad. But for us, it's essential that in pursuing a healthy weight, you maintain the joy of food. That's why we were delighted when we realized that Sirtfoods and the foods that enhance their action like protein and omega-3 food sources are prepared to fulfill our taste desire. It's the ultimate win-win: The Sirtfood diet is boosting our health and great tastes.

Let's go back one step and see how this works. Our taste buds determine how delicious we find our food, and how satisfied we are to eat it. This is done by seven major receptors to the taste. Human beings have evolved over countless generations to seek out the tastes that stimulate these receptors to achieve maximum nutrition out of our diet. The more those taste receptors are activated by a portion of food, the more satisfaction we get from a meal. And we have the ultimate menu in the Sirtfood Diet for happy taste buds, because it offers maximum stimulation across all taste receptors. To summarize these tastes and the foods you'll eat on the diet that satisfy them: the seven major sensations of taste are sweet (strawberries, dates); salty (celery, fish); sour (strawberries); bitter (cocoa, kale, endive, extra virgin olive oil, green tea); pungent (chilies, garlic, extra virgin olive oil); astringent (green tea, red wine); and umami (soy, fish, meat).

What we have discovered is that the greater a food's sirtuin-activating properties, the stronger it stimulates those taste centers and the more gratification we get from the food we eat. Importantly, it also ensures our hunger is fulfilled quicker, and our ability to consume more is that accordingly. That is a key reason why those following a Sirtfood-rich diet are faster pleasantly fuller.

Natural cocoa, for example, has a striking, appealing bitter taste, but remove the sirtuin-activating flavanols with aggressive industrial food processing techniques, and we're left with mass-produced, bland, and characterless cocoa that is used to make highly sweetened chocolate pastries. The health benefits have faded by this point.

The same is true of olive oil. Consumed in its minimally processed form — extra virgin — it has a strong and distinct taste that can be felt at the back of the throat with a hard blow. Yet refined and processed olive oil loses all character, is mild and bland, and does not carry a kick like this. Similarly, hot chilies hold much more sirtuin-activating credentials than the milder varieties, and wild strawberries are much more tasteful than farmed ones due to richer sirtuin-activating nutrient content.

Not only that, but we also note that individual Sirtfoods can activate several receptors of taste: green tea is both bitter and astringent, and strawberries combine sweet and sour flavors. Initially, some palates won't get used to any of these flavors — so much of our western food is deprived of both nutrition and true taste — but you'll be surprised at how easily you develop affection for them. After all, humans have evolved to search for a diet rich in Sirtfoods, alongside balanced protein and omega-3 fatty acids, to fulfill our appetite's essential needs and, in effect, our health. This evolutionary cycle has been going on for centuries without us understanding the reasons, and it has ensured that we get the full benefit from eating these foods.

Embrace Eating

Let's give an experiment a try. We just want you to do us one very easy thing: don't worry about a white bear. What did you think? Of course a white bear. Why? For what? Because we told you they didn't. Don't tell us you're already there!

This was the trailblazing experiment conducted by psychology professor Daniel Wegner in 1987 that demonstrated that forced suppressing of thoughts induces a paradoxical and detrimental increase of how much we actually think about what we are attempting to suppress. This is because instead of removing it from our minds, the attempt creates a fixation with the suppressed thought.

And as you've probably guessed, this phenomenon doesn't just apply to white bears. The exact same thing happens when we are making villains and restricting weight loss foods. Studies show that, in fact, we think more often about them, increasing the temptation. It's eating away before we eat it! And now we are much more likely to binge with the diet broken and the heightened anxiety about the "forbidden" things we have experienced.

Now the scientists have explained what's going on here. We just need to be fully autonomous. When we feel restricted, like going on a strict diet, this creates a negative atmosphere, which makes us feel uncomfortable. We feel caught up in this negativity, and we rebel to break out. We protest by doing what we've been told we shouldn't be doing, and doing it a lot more than we should have at first. It happens to us all, even to the most self-controlled ones. It's not a question of when but if. Scientists now believe that this is a critical reason why we can maintain diets and even see initial results but fail to see long-term success.

So does this mean that there is no point in even trying to alter our eating habits? Are we just doomed to fail? No, it means that we need to make our own optimistic, desired decision when making a change to be successful. We now know that it is not through dietary exclusion but through dietary inclusion that we can achieve that. Instead of focusing your energy on the negatives of what you shouldn't eat, instead, focus on the positive aspects of what you should eat. You avoid the psychological reaction by doing so. And the Sirtfood Diet's beauty is this. It's about what you put in your diet and not what you're taking out. It's about the quality and not the quantity of your food. And it's about you wanting to do it because you feel satisfied eating great-tasting foods with the additional knowledge that every bite provides a bounty of advantages.

Most diets constitute a means to an end. They're about hanging in there, trying to keep sight of the "thin ideal." But, at the end of the day, that rarely comes before the diet fails, and it's rarely sustained, even if achieved. There's a particular Sirtfood Diet. It's all about flying. Phase 1, which limits calories, is kept intentionally short and sweet to ensure motivating results are finished before any negative backlash occurs. The focus then is exclusively on Sirtfoods. And the desire to eat Sirtfoods isn't just motivated by an end result of weight loss. Rather it is just as much if not more about appreciating and enjoying real food for a healthy, fit lifestyle.

What's more, once you reap Sirtfoods' unique benefits, from satisfying your appetite to enhancing your quality of life, you'll find your habits and tastes change. With the Sirtfood Diet, foods that would have previously set off the cascade of negative reactions if you were told that you couldn't eat them will lose their appeal and diminish their hold over you. They become a minor part of your diet, and they all reached without a single white bear sighting.

Let's Wrap This Up!

- The Sirtfood Diet takes the world's most potent sirtfoods and brings them together in a simple and practical way to eat.
- In order to achieve optimum results in terms of weight loss and health, Sirtfoods should be eaten in the right quantity, combination, and forms to reap the synergistic benefits of their sirtuin-activating compounds.
- We further improve this by adding other healthy ingredients such as leucine-rich protein foods and oily fish, to make the Sirtfood Diet's effects even more potent.
- Eating earlier in the day is also vital and helps to keep us in sync with our built-in body clock.
- In comparison to our western diets, Sirtfoods satisfy all of our taste receptors, meaning we get more satisfaction from our food and feel satisfied faster.
- Sirtfood diet is an inclusion diet – not an exclusion diet, making it the only form of diet that can offer long-term weight-loss results.

CHAPTER SIX: TOP 20 SIRTFOODS

Now that you know everything about Sirtfoods, why they're so powerful, and what it takes to create an effective diet that will deliver lasting results, it's time to get started. The next chapter marks the start of day one of the Sirtfood Diet. So this is the perfect time to get acquainted with each of the top twenty Sirtfoods, which will soon become the staples of your daily diet.

Arugula

Clearly, Arugula (also known as rocket, rucola, rugula, and roquette) has a colorful background in American food culture. A pungent green salad leaf with a distinctive peppery taste, it quickly ascended from humble roots as the basis of many Mediterranean peasant dishes to become a symbol of food snobbery in the United States, even leading to the coining of the term arugulance!

But long before it was a salad leaf wielded in a war of class, arugula was revered for its medicinal properties by the ancient Greeks and Romans. Commonly used as a diuretic and digestive aid, it gained its true fame from its reputation for having potent aphrodisiac properties, so much so that the growth of arugula was banned in monasteries in the Middle Ages, and the famous Roman poet Virgil wrote that "the rocket excites the sexual desire of drowsy people." A combination of kaempferol and quercetin is being investigated as a cosmetic ingredient in addition to powerful sirtuin-activating properties because together, they moisturize and enhance collagen synthesis in the skin. With those credentials, it's time to drop any elitist tag and make this the leaf of choice for salad bases, where it perfectly pairs with an extra virgin olive oil dressing, combining to do a potent double act of Sirtfood

Buckwheat

Buckwheat was one of Japan's first domesticated crops, and the story goes that when Buddhist monks made long trips into the mountains, they'd only bring a cooking pot and a buckwheat bag for food. Buckwheat is so nutritious that this was all they needed, and it fed them up for weeks. We're huge fans of buckwheat too. Firstly, because it is one of a sirtuin activator's best-known sources, called rutin. But also because it has advantages as a cover crop, improving soil quality and suppressing weed growth, making it a fantastic crop for environmentally sound and sustainable agriculture.

One reason buckwheat is head and shoulders above other, more popular grains is possibly because it's not a grain at all — it's actually a rhubarb-related fruit seed. Having one of the highest protein content of any grain, as well as being a Sirtfood powerhouse, makes it an unrivaled alternative to more widely used grains. Moreover, it is as versatile as any grain, and being naturally gluten-free, it is a great choice for those intolerant to gluten.

Capers

In case you're not so familiar with capers, we're talking about those salty, dark green, pellet-like things on top of a pizza that you may only have had occasion to see. Yet surely, they are one of the most undervalued and overlooked foods out there. Intriguingly, they are actually the caper bush's flower buds, which grow abundantly in the Mediterranean before being picked and preserved by hand. Studies now reveal that capers possess important antimicrobial, antidiabetic, anti-inflammatory, immunomodulatory, and antiviral properties, and have a rich history of being used as a medicine in the Mediterranean and North Africa. It's hardly surprising when we discover that they are crammed with nutrients that activate sirtuin.

We think it is about time these tiny morsels had their share of glory, so often overshadowed by the other heavy hitters from the Mediterranean diet. Flavor-wise it's a case of big stuff coming in small packages, as they're sure they're punching. But if you don't know how to use them, then don't feel intimidated. For these diminutive nutrient superstars, which combined with the right ingredients provide a beautifully distinctive and inimitable sour/salty flavor to round off a dish in style, we'll soon have you up to speed and falling head over heels.

Celery

For millennia, Celery was around and revered — with leaves found adorning the remains of the Egyptian pharaoh

Tutankhamun who died around 1323 BCE. Early strains were very bitter, and celery was generally considered a medicinal plant, especially for cleansing and detoxification to prevent disease. This is especially interesting considering that liver, kidney, and gut safety are among the many promising benefits that science is now showing. In the seventeenth century, it was domesticated as a vegetable, and selective breeding reduced its strong bitter flavor in favor of sweeter varieties, thus establishing its place as a traditional salad vegetable.

It is important to note when it comes to celery, that there are two types: blanched/yellow and Pascal / green. Blanching is a technique developed to reduce the characteristic bitter taste of the celery, which has been perceived to be too strong. This involves shading the celery before harvesting from sunlight, resulting in a paler color and a milder flavor. What a travesty that is, for blanching dumbs down the sirtuin-activating properties of celery as well as dumbing down the flavor. Fortunately, the tide is changing, and people are demanding real and distinct flavor, turning back to the greener variety. Green celery is the sort that we suggest you use in both the green juices and meals, with the heart and leaves being the most nutritious pieces.

Chilies

Chili has been an integral part of the gastronomic experience worldwide for thousands of years. On one level, it's disconcerting that we'd be so enamored with it. Its pungent heat, triggered by a substance called capsaicin in chilies, is designed as a mechanism of plant defense to cause pain and dissuade predators from feasting on it, yet we appreciate that. The food and our infatuation with it are almost mystical. Incredibly, one study showed that eating chilies together even increases individual cooperation. And we know from a health perspective that their seductive heat is fantastic to activate our sirtuins and boost our metabolism. The culinary applications of the chili are also endless, making it a simple way to offer a hefty Sirtfood boost to any dish.

While we appreciate that not everyone is a fan of hot or spicy foods, we hope we can entice you to consider adding small amounts of chilies, especially in light of recent research showing that those eating spicy foods three or more times a week have a 14 percent lower death rate compared to those eating them less than once a week. The hotter the chili, the better its Sirtfood credentials, but be sensitive and stick with what suits your own tastes. Serrano peppers are a great start — they are tolerable for most people when packing heat, and for more experienced heat seekers, we suggest looking for optimum sirtuin-activating benefits for Thai chilies. It can be difficult to find in grocery stores, but they can also be sold in specialty markets in Asia. Opt for deep-colored peppers, avoiding those with a wrinkled and fuzzy appearance.

Cocoa

We saw the impressive health benefits of cocoa on pages 59–60, so it's no surprise to learn that cocoa was considered a sacred food for ancient civilizations like the Aztecs and Mayans, and was usually reserved for the elite and warriors, served at feasts to gain loyalty and duty. Indeed, there was such high regard for the cocoa bean that it was even used as a form of currency. It was commonly served as a frothy beverage back then. But what could be a more delicious way to get our dietary quota of cacao than through chocolate?

Unfortunately, there's no count here for the diluted, refined, and highly sweetened milk chocolate we commonly munch. We're talking about chocolate with 85 percent solids of cocoa to earn its Sirtfood badge. But even then, aside from the percentage of cocoa, not every chocolate is created equal. To reduce its acidity and give it a darker color, chocolate is often treated with an alkalizing agent (known as the Dutch process). Sadly, this process diminishes its sirtuin-activating flavanols massively, thereby seriously compromising its health-promoting quality. Fortunately, and unlike in many other countries, food labeling regulations in the United States require that alkalized cocoa must be declared as such and labeled "processed with alkali." We recommend avoiding these products, even if they boast a higher cocoa percentage, and instead opting for those that have not undergone Dutch processing to reap the true benefits of cocoa.

Coffee

What's all that about Sirtfood Coffee? We're listening to you. We can assure you that there is no typo. Gone are the days when a twinge of guilt needed to temper our enjoyment of coffee. The work is unambiguous: coffee is a bona fide food for wellbeing. Indeed it is a true treasure trove of fantastic nutrients that activate sirtuin. And with more than half of Americans consuming coffee every day (to the tune of $40 billion a year!), coffee enjoys the accolade of being America's number one source of polyphenols. The ultimate irony is that the one thing we were chastised by so many health "experts" for doing was, in fact, the best thing we were doing for our health each day. This is why coffee drinkers have slightly less diabetes, as well as lower levels of some cancers and neurodegenerative disease.

As for the ultimate irony, rather than being a poison, coffee actually strengthens our livers and makes them healthier! And contrary to the popular belief that coffee dehydrates the body, it is now well established not to be the case, with coffee (and tea) making a perfect contribution to the fluid intake of regular coffee drinkers. So while we appreciate that coffee is not for everybody and some people may be very sensitive to the effects of caffeine, it's happy days for those who enjoy a cup of coffee.

Virgin Olive Oil

Olive oil is the most renowned of Mediterranean traditional diets. The olive tree is among the world's oldest-known cultivated trees, also known as the "immortal tree." And since people began squeezing olives in stone mortars to gather them, the oil has been respected, almost 7,000 years ago. Hippocrates quoted it as a cure-all; now, a few millennia later, modern science unequivocally asserts its marvelous health benefits. There is now a plethora of scientific evidence showing that daily olive oil intake is highly cardioprotective, as well as playing a role in minimizing the risk of major modern-day diseases such as diabetes, other cancers, and osteoporosis, and associated with improved longevity.

When it comes to olive oil, the trick is to buy extra virgin to reap the goodness of Sirtfood in full. Virgin olive oil is only obtained from the fruit by mechanical means under conditions that do not contribute to the degradation of the oil, so the consistency and the polyphenol content can be guaranteed. "Extra virgin" refers to the first pressing of the fruit ("virgin" is the second pressing); it has the greatest taste, quality, and credentials of Sirtfood, and is, therefore, the one that we strongly recommend using.

Apple

Garlic has been considered one of Nature's wonder foods for thousands of years, with soothing and rejuvenating properties. Egyptians fed pyramid crews with garlic to enhance their immunity, avoid various diseases, and strengthen their performance through their ability to prevent fatigue. Garlic is a potent natural antibiotic and antifungal that is often used to help treat ulcers in the stomach. By accelerating the removal of waste products from the body, it can stimulate the lymphatic system to "detox" And as well as being investigated for fat loss, it also packs a potent heart health punch, lowering cholesterol by about 10 percent, and lowering blood pressure by 5 to 7 percent, as well as lowering blood stickiness and blood sugar levels.

And if you're worried about the off-putting garlic odor, note. When women were asked to evaluate a selection of men's body odors, those men who consumed four or more garlic cloves a day were judged to have a much more appealing and pleasant odor. Researchers believe this is because it is perceived as signaling better health. And there are always mints for fresher breath, of course!

Eating garlic has a trick to get maximum benefit. In garlic, the Sirtfood nutrients are complemented by another key nutrient in it called allicin, which gives off the characteristic aroma of garlic. But after physical "injury" to the bulb, allicin only occurs in garlic. And, when exposed to heat (cooking) or low pH (stomach acid), its formation is halted. So when preparing garlic, chop, thin, or crush, and then allow it to sit for about ten minutes before cooking or eating the allicin.

Green Tea (Matcha in particular),

Many will be familiar with green tea, the toast of the Orient, and ever more popular in the West. Like the growing awareness of its health benefits, green tea consumption is linked to less cancer, heart disease, diabetes, and osteoporosis. The reason it is thought that green tea is so good for us is primarily due to its rich content of a group of powerful plant compounds called catechins, the star of the show being a particular type of sirtuin-activating catechin known as epigallocatechin gallate (EGCG).

What's the fuss about matcha, though? We like to think of matcha on the steroids as normal green tea. In comparison to traditional green tea, which is prepared as an infusion, it is a special powdered green tea which is prepared by dissolving directly in water. The upshot of drinking matcha is that it contains significantly higher levels of the sirtuin-activating compound EGCG than other green tea forms. Zen priests describe matcha as the "ultimate mental and medical remedy [which] has the ability to make one's life more complete" if you are looking for further endorsement.

Kale

We are at heart cynics, so we are always skeptical about what drives the latest craze for superfood advertising. Is it science, or are its interests at stake? In recent years few foods have exploded as dramatically as kale on the health scene. Described as the "lean, green brassica queen" (referring to its cruciferous vegetable family), it has become the chic vegetable for which all health-lovers and foodies are gunning. Every October, there is even a National Day of the Kale. But you don't have to wait until then to show your kale pride: there are also T-shirts, with trendy slogans like "Powered by Kale" and "Highway to Kale." That's enough for us to set the alarm bells ringing.

We've done the research, filled with suspicions, and we have to admit that our conclusion is that kale really deserves her pleasures (although we still don't recommend the T-shirts!). The reason we're pro-kale is that it boasts bumper amounts of the quercetin and kaempferol sirtuin-activating nutrients, making it a must-include in the Sirtfood Diet and the base of our green Sirtfood juice. What's so refreshing about kale is that kale is available everywhere, locally grown, and very affordable, unlike the usual exotic, hard-to-source, and exorbitantly priced so-called superfoods!

Medjool Dates

It may come as a surprise to include Medjool dates in a list of foods that stimulate weight loss and promote health—especially when we tell you that Medjool dates contain a staggering 66 percent sugar. Sugar doesn't have any sirtuin-activating properties at all; rather, it has well-established links to obesity, heart disease, and diabetes — just the opposite of what we're looking to achieve. But processed and refined sugar is very different from sugar carried in a naturally supplied vehicle balanced with sirtuin-activating polyphenols: the date of the Medjool.

Medjool dates, consumed in moderation, in total contrast to regular sugar, do not really have any significant measurable impact on blood-sugar-raising. On the contrary, eating them is related to having less diabetes and heart disease. They have been a staple food worldwide for centuries, and in recent years there has been an explosion of scientific interest in dates that views them emerging as a potential medicine for a number of diseases. Here lies the uniqueness and power of the Sirtfood Diet: it refutes the dogma and allows you to indulge in sweet things in moderation without feeling guilty.

Parsley

Parsley is something of a culinary conundrum. It so often appears in recipes, yet so often it's the green token guy. At best, we serve a couple of chopped sprigs and tossed as an afterthought on a meal, at worst a solitary sprig for decorative purposes only. Either way, there on the plate, it is often still languishing long after we have finished eating. This culinary styling stems from its traditional use in ancient Rome as a garnish for eating after meals in order to refresh breath, rather than being part of the meal itself. And what a shame, because parsley is a fantastic food that packs a vibrant, refreshing taste full of character.

Taste aside, what makes parsley very unique is that it is an excellent source of the sirtuin-activating nutrient apigenin, a real blessing because it is rarely contained in other foods in large amounts. In our brains, apigenin binds fascinatingly to the benzodiazepine receptors, helping us to relax and help us to sleep. Stock it all up, and it's time we loved parsley not as omnipresent food confetti, but as a food in its own right to reap the wonderful health benefits that it can offer.

Red Endive

Endive is a fairly new kid on the block in so far as vegetables go. Tale has it that a Belgian farmer found endive in 1830, by mistake. The farmer stored chicory roots in his cellar, and then used them as a form of coffee substitute, only to forget them. Upon his return, he discovered that white leaves had sprouted, which he found to be tender, crunchy, and rather delicious upon degustation. Endive is now grown all over the world, including the USA, and earns its Sirtfood badge thanks to its impressive sirtuin activator luteolin content. And besides the established sirtuin-activating benefits, luteolin consumption has become a promising approach to therapy to improve sociability in autistic children.

It has a crisp texture and a sweet taste for those new to endive, followed by a gentle and friendly bitterness. If you're ever stuck on how to increase endive in your diet, you can't fail by adding her leaves to a salad where her warm, tart flavor adds the perfect bite to an extra virgin olive oil dressing based on zesty. Red is best, just like an onion, but the yellow variety can also be considered a Sirtfood. So while the red variety may sometimes be more difficult to find, you can rest assured that yellow is a perfectly appropriate alternative.

Red dumplings

Since the time of our prehistoric ancestors, onions have been a dietary staple, being one of the first crops to be grown, around 5,000 years ago. With such a long history of use and such strong health-giving properties, many cultures that came before us have revered onions. They were held especially by the Egyptians as objects of worship, regarding their circle-within-a-circle structure as symbolic of eternal life. And the Greeks believed that onions made athletes stronger. Athletes would eat their way through vast amounts of oignons before the Olympic Games, even drinking the juice!

It's an incredible testimony to how valuable ancient dietary wisdom can be when we consider that onions earn their top twenty Sirtfood status because they're chock-full of the sirtuin-activating compound quercetin — the very compound that the sports science world has recently started actively researching and marketing to improve sports performance. And why the red ones? Simply because they have the highest content of quercetin, although the standard yellow ones do not lag too far behind, and are also a good inclusion.

Red Wine

Any list of the top twenty Sirtfoods would not be complete without the incorporation of the original Sirtfood, red wine. The French paradox made headlines in the early 1990s, with it being discovered that despite the French appearing to do everything wrong when it came to health (smoking, lack of exercise, and rich food consumption), they had lower death rates from heart disease than countries like the United States. The reason for this was suggested by doctors was the copious amount of red wine consumed. Danish researchers then published work in 1995 to show that low-to-moderate consumption of red wine reduced death rates, whereas similar levels of beer alcohol had no effect, and similar intakes of hard liquors increased death rates. Obviously, in 2003, the rich content of red wine from a bevy of sirtuin-activating nutrients was discovered, and the rest, as they claim, was made history.

But there is even more to the impressive resume of red wine. Red wine appears to be able to ward off the common cold, with moderate wine drinkers having a reduction in its incidence of more than 40%. Studies now also show benefits for oral health and cavity prevention. With moderate consumption, social bonding, and out-of-the-box thinking have also been shown to increase, after-work drinks among colleagues appear to have been available to discuss work projects.

Moderation is, of course, key. For the gain from this, only small quantities are required, and excess alcohol easily undoes the nice. The sweet spot appears to stick up to one 5-ounce drink per day for women and up to two 5-ounce drinks per day for men according to US guidelines. Wines from the New York region (especially pinot noir, cabernet sauvignon, and merlot) have the highest polyphenol content of the most widely available wines to ensure maximum sirtuin-activating bang for your buck.

Soy

Soja products have a long history as an important part of many Asia-Pacific countries' diets, such as China, Japan, and Korea. Researchers first turned to soy after they discovered that high soy-consuming countries had significantly lower rates of certain cancers, particularly breast and prostate cancers. It is believed to be due to a special group of soybean polyphenols known as isoflavones, which can favorably affect how estrogens function in the body, including daidzein and sirtuin-activators of formononetin. Intake of soy products was also linked to a reduction in the frequency or severity of a variety of conditions such as cardiovascular disease, menopause symptoms, and bone loss.

Highly refined, nutrient-stripped types of soybean are a common component now added to many packaged foods. The benefits are reaped only from natural soy products such as tofu, an excellent source of vegan protein, or in a fermented form such as tempeh, natto, or our favorite, miso, a typical Japanese paste fermented with a naturally occurring fungus that results in an intense taste of umami.

Blueberries

In recent years, the fruit has become increasingly vilified, getting a bad rap in the growing fervor toward sugar. Fortunately, such a malignant image couldn't be more undeserved for berry-lovers. While all berries are powerhouses of nutrition, strawberries are winning their top twenty Sirtfood status due to their abundance of the fisetin sirtuin activator. And now studies support regular eating strawberries to promote healthy aging, staying off Alzheimer's, cancer, diabetes, heart disease, and osteoporosis. As for their sugar content, a mere teaspoon of sugar per three and a half ounces is very small.

Intriguingly and naturally low in sugar itself, strawberries have marked effects on how the body treats carbohydrates. What researchers have found is that adding strawberries to carbohydrates has the effect of reducing demand for insulin, essentially turning the food into a sustained energy releaser. And new research now suggests that eating strawberries has similar effects in diabetes treatment to drug therapy. William Butler, the great physician of the seventeenth century, wrote in praise of the strawberry: "Doubtless God could have made a better berry, but without a doubt, God never did." We can only agree.

Tumeric.

Turmeric, a cousin of ginger, is the new kid in food trends on the block, with Google naming it the ingredient of the 2015 breakout star. While we are just turning to it nowhere in the West, it has been valued for thousands of years in Asia, for both culinary and medical reasons. Incredibly, India is generating almost the entire world's turmeric supply, eating 80 percent of it itself. In addition to the benefits of the "golden spice", in Asia, turmeric is used to treat skin conditions like acne, psoriasis, dermatitis, and rash. Before Indian weddings, there is a ritual where the turmeric paste is applied as a skin beauty treatment to the bride and groom but also to symbolize the warding off evil.

One thing that limits turmeric's effectiveness is that its key sirtuin-activating nutrient, curcumin, is poorly absorbed by the body as we eat it. Research, however, shows that we can overcome this by cooking it in liquid, adding fat, and adding black pepper, all of which increase its absorption dramatically. This fits perfectly with traditional Indian cuisine, wherein curries and other hot dishes it is typically combined with ghee and black pepper, and yet again proves that science only catches up with the age-old wisdom of traditional eating methods.

Walnuts

Dating back to 7000 BCE, walnuts are the oldest known man-made tree food, originating in ancient Persia, where they were the preserve of royalty. Quick forward to the present day and walnuts are a success story in the US. California is leading the way, with California's Central Valley famous for being the prime walnut-growing region. California walnuts provide the United States with 99 percent of commercial supply and whopping three-quarters of worldwide walnut trade.

Walnuts lead the way as the number one nut for health, according to the NuVal system, which ranks foods according to how safe they are and has been endorsed by the American College of Preventive Medicine. But what really makes walnuts stand out for us is how they fly in the face of traditional thinking: they are high in fat and calories, but well-established for weight loss, and the risk of metabolic diseases like cardiovascular disease and diabetes is reduced. That is the strength of triggering the sirtuin.

The emerging research showing walnuts to be a powerful anti-aging food is less well known but equally intriguing. Research also points to their benefits as a brain food with the potential to slow down brain aging and reduce the risk of degenerative brain disorders, as well as preventing the decline in physical function wit

CHAPTER SEVEN: PHASE 1: LOSING 7 POUNDS IN SEVEN DAYS

Welcome to Sirtfood Diet, Phase 1. This is the phase of hyper-success, where you are going to take a huge step towards achieving a slimmer and leaner body. Follow our simple step-by-step instructions and use the delicious recipes you'll get. We also have a meat-free version in addition to our standard seven-day plan, which is suitable for vegetarians and vegans alike. Feel free to go along with whatever you like.

What to Expect

You'll enjoy the full benefits of our scientifically validated strategy of losing 7 pounds in seven days during Phase 1. But remember that includes gaining muscle, so don't just get hung up with the numbers on the scales. Nor should you become accustomed to weighing yourself daily. In addition, in the last few days of Phase 1, we sometimes see the scales rising due to muscle growth, while waistlines begin to shrink. Therefore, we want you to look at the scales, but not be governed by them. Find out how you look inside the mirror, how your clothes match, or whether you need to push a knot on your belt. These are all great indicators of the greater changes in your body makeup.

Be mindful of other improvements, too, such as well-being, energy levels, and how smooth the skin looks. At your local pharmacy, you can even get measurements of your overall cardiovascular and metabolic health to see changes in things like your blood pressure, blood sugar levels, and blood fats like cholesterol and triglycerides. Remember, weight loss aside, introducing Sirtfoods into your diet is a huge step in making your cells fitter and more disease resistant, setting you up for an exceptional healthy lifetime.

How to Start Phase 1

In order to make Phase 1 as plain sailing as possible, we will guide you one day at a time through the entire seven-day plan, including the lowdown on the Sirtfood green juice and easy-to-follow, delicious recipes every step of the way.

Phase 1 of the Sirtfood Diet consists of two distinct phases:

Days 1 to 3 are the most intensive and you can eat up to a limit of 1000 calories every day during this period, consisting of:

- 3 x Green Sirtfood juices
- 1 x main meal

Days 4 to 7 will see your daily intake of food grow to a limit of 1,500 calories, consisting of:

- 2 x Green Sirtfood juices
- 2 x Hauptgerichte

There are very few rules with which to follow the diet. Ultimately, for sustained success, it's about incorporating it into your lifestyle and around daily life. But here are a few simple yet big-impact tips to get the best result:

1. **Get a Good Juicer**: Juicing is an important part of the Sirtfood Diet, and a juicer is one of the best investments you'll make for your wellbeing. While the budget should be the determining factor, some juicers are more efficient at extracting the juice from green leafy vegetables and herbs, with the Breville brand among the best juicers we've tried.
2. **Preparation Is Key**: One thing is evident from the abundance of feedback we've had: the most effective were those who prepared ahead of time. Get to know the ingredients and recipes and stock up on what's needed. You'll be surprised at how simple the whole process is, with everything planned and ready.
3. **Save Time**: Prepare cleverly when you're tight on time. Meals can be rendered the previous night. Juices can be made in bulk and stored in the refrigerator for up to three days (or longer in the freezer) until their sirtuin-activating nutrient levels begin to fall. Just shield it from light, and add only when you're ready to eat it in the matcha.

4. **Eat Early**: Eating earlier in the day is better, and ideally, meals and juices should not be consumed later than 7 p.m, but in the end, the diet is tailored to suit the lifestyle and late eaters still benefit greatly.
5. **Space Out the Juices**: They should be consumed at least one hour before or two hours after a meal to enhance the absorption of green juices and spread throughout the day, rather than being too close together.
6. **Eat until Satisfied**: Sirtfoods can have a dramatic effect on appetite, and some people will be full before their meals are finished. Listen to your body and eat until satisfied, instead of forcing down all the food. Say, "Hara Hachi bu," as the long-lived Okinawans do, which roughly means "Eat until you're 80 percent full."
7. **Enjoy the Journey**: Don't get caught on the end goal, but stay mindful of the journey instead. This diet is about celebrating food in all its wonder, for its health benefits but also for the enjoyment and pleasure it brings. Research shows that we are far more likely to succeed if we keep our minds focused on the path rather than the final destination.

What to Drink

As well as the recommended daily servings of green juices, other fluids can be freely consumed throughout Phase 1. Non-calorie beverages, preferably plain juice, black coffee, and green tea. If your normal preferences are for black or herbal teas, do not hesitate to include these too. Fruit juices and soft drinks are left behind. Instead, try adding a few sliced strawberries to still or sparkling water to make your own Sirtfood-infused health drink, if you want to jazz things up. Keep it for a few hours in the fridge, and you will have a pleasantly refreshing alternative to soft drinks and juices.

One thing you ought to be mindful of is that we are not recommending any big abrupt changes in your everyday use of coffee. Symptoms of caffeine withdrawal may make you feel crappy for a couple of days; likewise, large rises can be painful for those particularly prone to caffeine effects. We also suggest drinking coffee without adding milk, as some researchers have found that the addition of milk can minimize the absorption of beneficial nutrients that activate sirtuin. The same was found for green tea, although adding some lemon juice actually increases the absorption of its nutrients, which activate sirtuin.

Remember, this is the hyper-success time, and while you might be comforted by the fact that it's only for a week, you need to be a little more vigilant. For this week, we have alcohol in the form of red wine but as a cooking ingredient only.

The Sirtfood Green Juice

The green juice is an integral component of the Sirtfood Diet's Phase 1 program. All the ingredients are strong Sirtfoods, and in every juice, you get a potent cocktail of natural compounds like apigenin, kaempferol, luteolin, quercetin, and EGCG that work together to turn on your sirtuin genes and promote fat loss. To that, we have added lemon, as it has been shown that its natural acidity protects, stabilizes, and increases the absorption of the sirtuin-activating nutrients. We added a touch of apple and ginger to taste too. So, both of these are optional. Yes, many people notice that they leave the apple out entirely until they become used to the taste of the fruit.

GREEN JUICE SIRTFOOD (SERVES 1)

- 2 Strong handfuls (approximately 21/2 ounces, or 75 g)
- A big handful of arugula (1 ounce or 30 g)
- A very small handful of flat-leaf parsley (about 1/4 ounce, or 5 g)
- 2 to 3 wide stalks of celery (51/2 ounces or 150 g), including the leaves
- 1/2 Medium Apple Green
- Fresh ginger 1/2- to 1-inch (1-2.5 cm)
- 1/2 lemon juice
- Matcha powder at 1/2 teaspoon level (optional)

Phase 1 to 3 days: Added only to the first two juices of the day;

Phase 1 Days 4 to 7: Added in both juices

- Notice that while we weighed all the quantities exactly as described in our pilot trial, our experience is that a handful of measures work extremely well. In fact, they are better at tailoring the number of nutrients to the body size of an individual. Larger people tend to have larger hands, and thus get a proportionally higher amount of Sirtfood nutrients to match their body size, and vice versa for smaller people.
- Blend the greens together (kale, arugula, and parsley), then add the juice. We consider that juicers may really vary in their efficiency when juicing leafy vegetables, so before going on to the other ingredients, you can need to juice the remainder. The target is to end up with about 2 ounces of fluid, or about 1/4 cup (50ml) of green juice.
- Now celery, apple, and ginger tea.
- You can also peel the lemon and put it through the juicer, but we find it much easier to squeeze the lemon into the juice by hand. You should have around 1 cup (250ml) of juice in total by this point, maybe somewhat more.
- You only add the matcha when the juice is made and ready for serving. In a bowl, pour a small amount of water, then add the matcha, and stir vigorously with a fork or tablespoon. In the first two drinks of the day, we only use matcha, as it contains small levels of caffeine (the same content as a regular teacup). If drunk late, it can keep you awake for people not used to it.
- Add the remaining liquid until the matcha is dissolved. Give it a swirl end; then, your juice is ready to drink. Free to top up with plain water, as you like.

Step 1: Your Seven-Day Guide

Take the juices at separate times of the day for Days 1 to 3 (e.g., first thing in the morning, mid-morning and mid-afternoon), and select one of the standard or vegan meal options and eat them at a time that suits you (usually eaten for lunch or dinner).

Day One

You'll consume on Day 1:
- 3 x Green Sirtfood juices
- 1 x (standard or vegan option) main meal, either:

Stir-fry Asian shrimp with buckwheat noodles

+

Dark chocolate (85 percent cocoa solids) 1/2 to 3/4 ounce (15 to 20 g)

or

Miso and sesame glazed tofu with stir-fried green chili and ginger (vegan)

+

Dark chocolate (85 percent cocoa solids) 1/2 to 3/4 ounce (15 to 20 g)

Day two

You are going to eat on Day 2:
- 3 x Green Sirtfood juices
- 1 x (standard or vegan option) main meal, either:

Turkey's "couscous" spiced cauliflower with garlic, capers, and parsley

+

Dark chocolate (85 percent cocoa solids) 1/2 to 3/4 ounce (15 to 20 g)

or

Kale dal with buckwheat and red onion (vegan)

+

Dark chocolate (85 percent cocoa solids) 1/2 to 3/4 ounce (15 to 20 g)

Day Three

You'll consume on Day 3:
- 3 x Green Sirtfood juices
- 1 x (standard or vegan option) main meal, either:

Aromatic chicken breast with kale and red onions, chili and tomato salsa

+

Dark chocolate (85 percent cocoa solids) 1/2 to 3/4 ounce (15 to 20 g)

or

Harissa baked 'couscous' tofu with cauliflower (vegan)

+

Dark chocolate (85 percent cocoa solids) 1/2 to 3/4 ounce (15 to 20 g)

Take the juices at separate times of the day for Days 4 to 7 (e.g., the first juice either in the morning or mid-morning, the second mid-afternoon juice); select your meals from either standard or vegan options and eat them at the right time (usually eaten for breakfast/lunch and dinner). You may also continue to add dark chocolate (85 percent cocoa solids) in 1/2 to 3/4 ounces (15 to 20 g) each day, at your discretion, depending on your appetite.

Day four

You'll eat on Day 4:
- 2 x Green Sirtfood juices
- 2 x main meals (with regular or vegan option):

MEAL 1: Sirt muesli

MEAL 2: Caramelized endive pan-fried salmon fillet, arugula, and celery leaf salad

or

MEAL 1: muesli-sirt (vegan)

MEAL 2: Tuscan (vegan) bean stew

Day five

You'll consume on Day 5:
- 2 x Green Sirtfood juices
- 2 x main meals (with regular or vegan option):

MEAL 1: Buckwheat Tabbouleh strawberries

MEAL 2: Baked cod, miso-marinated with stir-fried greens and sesame

or

MEAL 1: Buckwheat tabbouleh strawberries (vegan)

MEAL 2: Soba (buckwheat noodles) in tofu, celery, and kale (vegan) miso broth;

Day Six

You'll eat on Day 6:
- 2 x Green Sirtfood juices
- 2 x main meals (with regular or vegan option):

MEAL 1: Super salad with sirt

MEAL 2: Beef grilled with red wine juice, rings of onions, kale of garlic and potatoes grilled with herbs or

MEAL 1: super salad lentil sirt (vegan)

MEAL 2: mole kidney bean with potato boiled (vegan)

Day Seven

You'll eat on Day 7:
- 2 x Green Sirtfood juices
- 2 x main meals (with regular or vegan option):

MEAL 1: omelet syrup

MEAL 2: Baked walnut and parsley pesto chicken breast and red onion salad

or

MEAL 1: Salad with Waldorf (vegan)

MEAL 2: Walnut and parsley pesto and tomato salad (vegan) roasted eggplant wedges

CHAPTER EIGHT: PHASE 2: MAINTENANCE

Congratulations on concluding Sirtfood Diet Phase 1! You should already see great results with a fat loss and not only look slimmer and more toned but also feel revitalized and re-energized. So, now what? Having seen these often remarkable transformations ourselves firsthand, we know how much you're going to want to see even better results, not just preserve all those benefits. Sirtfoods are, after all, designed to eat for life. The question is how you customize what you did in Phase 1 into your usual dietary routine. That is exactly what prompted us to create a fourteen-day maintenance plan designed to help you make the transition from Phase 1 to your more normal dietary routine, thereby helping to sustain and extend the benefits of the Sirtfood Diet further.

What to Expect

You will maintain your weight loss results during Phase 2, and continue to lose weight gradually. Remember, the one striking thing we've found with the Sirtfood Diet is that most or all of the weight people lose is from fat and that many actually put some muscle in. So we would like to remind you again not to judge your progress purely on the scale by the numbers. Look in the mirror to see if you look leaner and more toned, see how well your clothes fit, and lap up the compliments you'll get from others.

Also remember that as the weight loss continues, so will the health benefits. By following the 14-day maintenance plan, you are really starting to lay the foundations for a lifelong healthy future.

How to Follow Phase 2

The secret to success in this process is having your diet packed full of Sirtfoods. To make it as easy as possible, we have prepared a seven-day menu plan for you to follow, including delicious family-friendly recipes, packed with Sirtfoods every day to the rafters (although see page 149 for children's advice). All you need to do is repeat the Seven Day Plan twice to complete Phase 2's fourteen days.

Your dict will consist of: for every fourteen days,
- 3 x Sirtfood-rich meals
- 1 x Sirtfood green Juice
- 1 to 2 x Sirtfood bite snacks on choice

Again, when you have to eat those, there are no strict rules. Be flexible around your day and fit them. Two simple thumb-rules are:
- Get your green juice either early in the morning, at least 30 minutes before breakfast, or in the middle of the morning.
- Try your best to eat your dinner by 7 p.m.

Portion Sizes

During Step 2, our attention is not on calorie counting. For the average citizen, this is not a realistic solution or even a good one in the long term. Rather we focus on sensible portions, really well-balanced meals, and most importantly, filling up on Sirtfoods so that you can continue to benefit from their fat-burning and health-promoting effects.

We've also designed the meals in the plan to make them satiate, making you feel satisfied for longer. That, combined with Sirtfoods' natural appetite-regulating effects, means you're not going to spend the next 14 days feeling hungry, but rather pleasantly satisfied, well-fed, and extremely well-nourished. Just like in Phase 1, remember to listen and be guided by your appetite. If you prepare meals according to our instructions and find that you are comfortably full before you finish a meal, then stop eating is perfectly fine!

Drinks

Throughout Phase 2, you'll continue to include one green juice daily. This is to hold your top with high Sirtfoods rates. Just as in Phase 1, you can freely absorb other fluids in Phase 2. Our favorite beverages include remaining plain water, homemade flavored water, coffee, and green tea. If black or white tea is your predilection, feel free to indulge. The same holds for herbal teas. The great thing is that during Phase 2, you will enjoy the occasional glass of red wine. Due to its content of sirtuin-activating polyphenols, especially resveratrol and piceatannol, red wine is a sirtfood which makes it by far the best choice of alcoholic beverage. However, with alcohol itself having harmful effects on our fat cells, restraint is always best, so we recommend restricting the consumption to one glass of red wine with a meal for two or three days a week in Phase 2.

Returning To Three Meals

You consumed just one or two meals per day during Phase 1, which gave you plenty of flexibility when you ate your meals. As we are now returning to a more normal routine and the time-tested pattern of three meals a day, talking about breakfast is a good time.

Eating a healthy breakfast sets us ready for the day, raising our levels of strength and focus. Eating earlier keeps our blood sugar and fat levels in check, in terms of our metabolism. That breakfast is a good thing is borne out by a number of studies, typically showing that people who eat breakfast regularly are less likely to overweight.

This is because of our internal body clocks. Our bodies are expecting us to eat early in anticipation of when we will be most busy and need food. Yet, as many as a third of us will skip breakfasts on any given day, it's a common symptom of our chaotic everyday life, and the impression is there's just not enough time to eat well. But as you will see, nothing could be further from the truth with the nifty breakfasts that we have laid out here for you. Whether it's the Sirtfood smoothie that can be drunk on the go, the premade Sirt muesli, or the quick and easy Sirtfood scrambled eggs/tofu, finding those extra few minutes in the morning will reap dividends not only for your day but also for your weight and health over the longer term.

With Sirtfoods working to overcharge our energy levels, there's, even more, to gain from getting a hit from them early in the morning to start your day. This is done not only by eating a Sirtfood-rich meal but above all, by consuming the green juice, which we suggest you have either first thing in the morning — at least thirty minutes before a meal — or mid-morning. We get a lot of reports from our own clinical experience of people who first drink their green juice and don't feel hungry for a few hours afterward. If this is the effect it's having on you, waiting a few hours before having breakfast is perfectly fine. Just don't skip this one. Alternatively, with a good breakfast, you can kick off your day, then wait two or three hours to have the green juice. Be versatile, and simply go for something that works for you.

CHAPTER NINE: SIRTFOODS FOR LIFE

Congratulations, both phases of the Sirtfood Diet have now stopped! Only let's take stock of what you have accomplished. You've completed the hyper-success phase, experiencing weight loss in the region of 7 pounds, which probably includes some desirable gain in muscle. You have consolidated that weight loss throughout the fourteen-day maintenance phase and further improved your body composition. Most importantly, you have marked the beginning of your own personal revolution in health. You took a stand against the tide of ill health, which strikes so often as we get older. The vision you have chosen for yourself is increased strength, vitality, and health.

By now, you'll be familiar with the top twenty Sirtfoods, and you've come to appreciate how powerful they are. Not only that, but you'll also have become quite adept at including them in your diet and enjoying them. For the continued weight loss and health they offer, it is important that these foods remain a prominent feature of your everyday eating routine. But still, they're just twenty foods, and after all, the spice of life is variety. What next, then?

We'll give you the blueprint for lifelong health in this chapter. It's about keeping the body in good condition with a healthy and safe diet for all and having all the health-enhancing nutrients that we need. It's about keeping on reaping the Sirtfood Diet's weight-loss rewards using the very best foods nature has to offer.

Beyond The Top Twenty Sirtfoods

We've seen why Sirtfoods are so beneficial: some plants have sophisticated stress-response systems that produce compounds that activate sirtuins — the same fasting and exercise-activated fat-burning and longevity system in the body. The greater the quantity of these compounds produced by plants in response to stress, the greater the benefit we derive from their feeding. Our list of the top twenty Sirtfoods is made up of the foods that really stand out because they are particularly packed full of these compounds, and hence the foods that have the most exceptional ability to impact body composition and wellbeing. But foods' sirtuin-activating effects aren't a concept of everything or nothing.

There are many other plants out there that contain moderate amounts of sirtuin-activating nutrients, and by consuming these liberally, we encourage you to really increase the range and diversity of your diet. The Sirtfood Diet is all about inclusion and the variety of sirtuin-activating foods that can be incorporated into the diet, especially if that means you can reap from your meals even more of your favorite foods to maximize pleasure and enjoyment.

Let's use the workout analogy. The top twenty Sirtfoods are the (much more pleasurable) equivalent of sweating it out at the gym, with Phase 1 being the "boot camp." By contrast, eating those other foods with more moderate levels of sirtuin-activating nutrients is like reaping the rewards of going out for a good walk. Compare that to the typical diet that has a nutritional value equivalent to lying all day on the couch watching TV. Sure, sweating it out in the gym is good, but if that is all you do, you will soon get fed up with it. That walk should also be encouraged, especially if it means that you don't instead choose to lie on the couch.

For example, in our top twenty Sirtfoods, we have included strawberries because they are the most notable source of the sirtuin activator fisetin. Yet if we look more closely at berries as a food category, we find that they have metabolic health benefits as well as safe aging. Reviewing their nutritional composition, we find that other berries such as blackberries, black currants, blueberries, and raspberries also have notable levels of nutrients that activate sirtuins.

The same remains true with nuts. Notwithstanding their calorific content, nuts are so effective that they positively encourage weight loss and help move inches from the waist. It is in addition to reducing chronic disease risk. Although walnuts are our champion nut, nutrients that activate sirtuin can also be found in chestnuts, pecans, pistachios, and even peanuts.

Then, we turn our attention to the grain. In recent years there has been, in some quarters, a growing aversion to grains. Studies, however, link whole grain consumption with decreased inflammation, diabetes, heart disease, and cancer. Although they do not rival the pseudo-grain buckwheat Sirtfood credentials, we do see the presence of significant sirtuin-activating nutrients in other whole grains. And needless to say, their sirtuin-activating nutrient content is decimated when whole grains are processed into refined "white" versions. These refined versions are quite the toxic bunch and are involved in a multitude of state-of-the-art health problems. We're not suggesting you should never eat them, but instead, you're going to be much better off sticking to the whole-grain variety wherever possible.

Quinoa is a strong Sirtfood choice for those wishing to remain gluten-free. And look no further than popcorn for a great, whole grain Sirtfood snack that everyone loves. With the likes of goji berries and chia seeds having Sirtfood properties, also notorious "superfoods" get on the board. That is most likely the unwitting reason for the health benefits they have observed. While it does mean that they are good for us to eat, we also know that there are cheaper, more accessible, and better options out there, so don't feel compelled to jump on that particular bandwagon! We see the same trend across a lot of food classes. Unsurprisingly, the foods that science has developed are generally healthy for us, and we should be consuming more of them. Below we listed another forty foods that we discovered have Sirtfood properties too. We strongly encourage you to incorporate these foods in order to sustain and continue your weight loss and health when you further broaden your diet repertoire.

Veggies

- Artichokes
- Asparagus
- Broccoli
- Green Drinks
- Shallots
- Watercress
- White Onions
- Yellow endive

Fruits

- Apples
- Blackberries
- Black currants
- Black Plums
- Cranberries
- Goji berries
- Kumquats
- Red grapes
- Raspberries

Nut and vegetables

- Chestnuts
- Chia seeds
- Peanuts
- Pecan nuts
- Pistachio nuts

Pseudo-seeds and seeds

- Maize popcorn
- Quinoa
- All-wheat flour
- Boobs fava
- White beans (for example, cannellini or navy);

Herbs and spices

- Chives
- Cinnamon
- Fresh and dried dill
- Dried orégano
- Dried sage
- Ginger
- Fresh and dried peppermint,
- Fresh and dried thyme;

Beverages

- Black Tea
- White   t

Protein Power

A high protein diet is one of the most popular diets of the last few years. Higher protein consumption when dieting has been found to promote satiety, maintain metabolism, and reduce muscle mass loss. But it's when they combine Sirtfoods with protein that things get taken to a whole new level.

Protein is, as you might remember, a necessary inclusion in a diet focused on Sirtfood to reap full benefits. Protein consists of amino acids, and it is a specific amino acid, leucine, which powerfully complements Sirtfoods' actions, enhancing their effects. This is done primarily by changing our cellular environment so that our diet's sirtuin-activating nutrients work much more effectively. This means we get the best result from a Sirtfood-rich meal, which is combined with protein-rich in leucine. Leucine's best dietary sources include red meat, poultry, fish, seafood, eggs, and dairy products.

Animal Protein

Animal products have been implicated in recent years as a contributing cause of many Western diseases, particularly cancer. If that really is the case, eating them with Sirtfoods may not sound like such a good idea. Here's our lowdown to lay that to rest. One of the major concerns about milk is that it is not just a simple food but a highly sophisticated signaling mechanism to induce rapid offspring body development. Although this has a valued purpose in early life, it may not be so appropriate in adult life. Persistent and hyperactivation of the key growth signal that dairy triggers in the body (called mTOR) are now associated with aging and the development of age-related disorders such as obesity, type 2 diabetes, cancer, and neurodegenerative diseases.1 Although the intricacies of this signaling system are a relatively new area of research, and thus still very much an unknown and theoretical risk, this is the case. However, evidence points to one thing: if we add Sirtfoods to a dairy-based diet, they inhibit the inappropriate effects of mTOR on our cells, revoke this risk and make Sirtfoods a must-include with a dairy-based diet.

Overall, reviews of the link between dairy and cancer are mixed. In the context of a Sirtfood rich diet, when we stack up all the research, moderate dairy consumption is perfectly fine and can offer many valuable nutrients to complement Sirtfoods.

As well as being a good source of protein, milk is an excellent source of vitamins and minerals, including iodine, calcium, and phosphorus. Our recommendation for adults is to eat up to three portions of milk (but not more than one quarter [1 liter] of milk or equivalent) every day. Poultry is perfectly safe when it comes to meat and cancer risk, but red and refined meats are even more suspect. Although evidence involving them in breast and prostate cancer on the ground is pretty poor, there is a serious concern that red and processed meat intake plays a role in intestinal cancer.6 Processed meat, such as ham, hot dogs, and pepperoni, tends to be the worst offender. While there is no need to completely strike it off the menu, it should be included in only small amounts, rather than being a staple.

The good news about red meat is that research shows that cooking it with Sirtfoods rescues the risk of cancer, whether it's making a marinade with herbs, spices, and extra virgin olive oil; cooking your beef with onions, or simply adding a nice cup of green tea to the meal or indulging in dark chocolate after dinner. These all pack a Sirtfood punch that actually helps neutralize the harmful effects of red meat. While we're all here to have your steak and eat it, don't go overboard. Red meat intake is best kept below about 1 pound (500 g) per week (cooked weight), roughly equivalent to 1.5 pounds (700 to 750 g) raw.

Poultry, along with vitamins and minerals such as vitamins B, potassium, and phosphorus, is an excellent source of protein. To adults, our advice is to eat it openly.

Red meat is also an excellent protein source, along with vitamins and minerals like iron, zinc, and vitamin B12. Our advice to adults is to eat up to three portions a week at most.

The link between egg consumption and cancer risk has not been investigated as extensively as meat and dairy products have, but there seems little reason for concern in this regard. What eggs have been involved in causing is heart disease, instead. This is because they represent a major dietary cholesterol source. Thus we are told to limit the use of eggs. It is interesting to note that other countries, including Nepal, Thailand, and South Africa, recommend egg consumption for their nutritional benefits as often as they do every day. Who is right, then? The evidence to siding with the latter is convincing. Regular consumption of eggs is not related to an increased risk of coronary heart disease or stroke. While particular genetic disorders may require a decreased intake of dietary cholesterol, this limitation is not important for the general population.

In addition to being a valuable source of protein, eggs are an excellent source of essential nutrients, such as vitamins B, vitamin A, and carotenoids. As part of a balanced diet, our recommendation for adults is to eat as desired.

The Power of Omega 3

The omega-3 long-chain fatty acids EPA and DHA are the second major group of nutrients that effectively complement Sirtfoods. Omega-3s have been the cherished nutritional health world favorite for years. What we didn't know before, which we are doing now, is that they also increase the activity of a subset of sirtuin genes in the body that is directly linked to longevity. This makes them the perfect match for Sirtfoods.

Omega-3s have beneficial effects in reducing inflammation and increasing fat blood levels. To that, we can add other heart-healthy effects: making the blood less likely to clot, stabilizing the heart's electrical rhythm, and reducing blood pressure. Even the pharmaceutical industry now turns to them as an aid in the fight against cardiac disease. And this is not where the litany of benefits stops. Omega-3s can have an impact on the way we think, having been shown to boost the mood and help stave off dementia.

When we talk about omega-3s, we're talking essentially about eating fish, especially oily varieties, because no other dietary source comes close to providing the significant levels of EPA and DHA that we need. And to see the benefits, all we need is two servings of fish a week, with an emphasis on oily fish. Unfortunately, the United States is not a nation of big fish eaters, and that is achieved by fewer than one in five Americans. As a result, our intake of the precious EPA and DHA is appallingly short.

Plant foods like nuts, beans, and green leafy vegetables often contain omega-3 but in a form called alpha-linolenic acid, which must be processed into EPA or DHA in the body. This conversion process is poor, meaning that alpha-linolenic acid delivers a negligible amount of our needs for omega-3. Even with the magnificent benefits of Sirtfoods, we shouldn't overlook the added value that consuming enough omega-3 fats brings. Within that order, the best sources of omega-3 fish are herring, sardines, salmon, trout, and mackerel. Although fresh tuna is naturally high too, the tinned variety loses the majority of the omega-3. And a supplement of DHA-enriched microalgae (up to 300 milligrams a day) is also recommended for vegetarians and vegans, though plant sources should still be integrated into the diet.

Oily fish, as well as being a valuable source of omega-3 and protein, is an excellent source of vitamins and minerals such as vitamins A and D, vitamins B, and trace minerals, including iodine and zinc. For adults, the recommendation is to eat at least two portions of fish, one of which is oily fish every week.

Can A Sirtfood Diet Provide All Of These?

To date, our focus has been solely on Sirtfoods and harvesting their maximum benefits to achieve the body we want and powerfully boosting our health in the process. But should that be a responsible, long-term dietary approach? After all, there is more to diet than mere sirtuin-activating nutrients. What about all the vitamins, minerals, and fibers that are also important for our well-being and the foods we can eat in order to meet those demands?

What we find intriguing is that if we keep a strong focus on Sirtfoods, supplemented by protein-rich foods and omega-3 sources, dietary needs are met across the whole spectrum of essential nutrients — much more so than any other diet, in fact. For example, we include kale because it is a powerful sirt food, but it is also a great source of minerals like vitamins C and K, folate and manganese, calcium, and magnesium. Kale is also a significant source of lutein and zeaxanthin carotenoids, both of which are important for eye protection, as well as immune-strengthening beta-carotene.

Walnuts also abound in minerals such as magnesium, copper, zinc, manganese, calcium, iron, and fiber. Buckwheat is packed with manganese, magnesium, copper, potassium, and fiber. Check vitamin B6, folate, potassium, and fiber ointment tubes. And strawberries are excellent sources of vitamin C as are potassium and manganese. And so it goes on.

Once you expand your diet to include the extended Sirtfood list and keep room for all the other good foods you unwittingly enjoy eating, what you'll end up with is a diet that's far richer in vitamins, minerals, and fiber than you've ever had before. In reality, what Sirtfoods offers is a missing category of food that changes the landscape of how we judge how healthy food is for us, and how we eat a genuinely full diet.

Rounding Out Diets Based On Plants

Sirtfoods is a celebration of the best vegetable foods in the world. Therefore, it should come as no surprise that vegetarians, who obviously have more in their diet, have reported lower levels of cancer, diabetes, heart disease, and obesity. Organizations such as the prestigious Academy of Nutrition and Dietetics are vociferous in their advocacy of vegetarian diets, arguing that they are healthy and nutritionally adequate, and in the prevention and treatment of many diseases may provide health benefits. Plant-based cooking is worthy of its own pleasures and worthy of a place for everyone at the dinner table. You must have seen this for yourself, like dishes like Butternut Squash and Date Tagine with Phase 2 Buckwheat for vegetarians and carnivores alike, offering their finest plant-based cuisine.

However, it is a different matter when it comes to eating vegan diets based solely on plants. The diet may turn out to be short, as Sirtfoods is good. Complementing Sirtfoods is a risk of nutritional deficiencies, without animal protein. We have already seen how essential fatty acids of omega-3 are for health and how plant sources are lacking. So our advice is to take a daily intake of DHA-enriched microalgae for vegetarians and vegans.

There is also a lack of vitamin B12 among vegetarians and particularly vegans. We can only get vitamin B12 from animal products (including dairy and eggs), so eat nothing but vegetable foods, and sooner or later, you will wind up deficient. If we are deficient in vitamin B12, we are exposed to an increased risk of heart disease, anemia, mental degeneration, depression, and dementia. When you want to eat a strictly plant-based diet, the best way around this conundrum is to take vitamin B12 in the form of an extra.

Another essential resource vegetables need to be mindful of calcium: the rate of vegetable fractures is 30 percent higher due to insufficient calcium intake. Although calcium can be obtained from a plant-based diet, a conscious effort is needed. Healthy sources of calcium in plants include green vegetables (e.g., kale, broccoli, bok choy), calcium-fortified drinks (soy milk, almond milk, rice milk), calcium tofu collection, nuts, and seeds. Even so, a moderate calcium supplement may still be required.

Ultimately, very high levels of iodine deficiency (80 percent in vegans and 25 percent in vegetarians) were found in people who consume diets based solely on plants. Iodine is essential for the development of thyroid hormones, which are completely crucial to the control of metabolism. Vegans run into trouble, with fish, meat, and milk being the dietary sources. Fortunately, iodized salt consumption is a simple way to increase the rate of iodine and is readily available in grocery stores. But for vegans that do not use an appreciable amount of iodized salt, a supplement is likely required. Although seaweed is a very rich source of iodine, it may contain extremely high and potentially excessive levels, which are just as bad for the thyroid as having too little and should not be relied on.

The Physical Activity Effect

The Sirtfood Diet is about eating those foods that are designed to promote sustained weight loss and well-being by nature. Even with the advantages that you see from adopting the diet, you can slip into the pit of feeling there's no need to exercise. This will be endorsed by many diet books, saying how ineffective exercise is compared with following the right diet for weight loss. And it's real; we can't outdo a bad diet. It's not the way we saw earlier that was intended to drive weight loss. It's inefficient, and the harmfulness of being too many borders. So it's true that till we see stars or achieve an Olympian's feats, there's no need to pound the treadmill — but what about general daily movement?

The fact is we are now much less active than we used to be. The age of technology has meant physical activity is virtually factored out of our daily lives, for all the advances it has brought. We don't really have to bother with the whole business of being active unless we actually want to. We can roll out of bed, drive to work, take the elevator, sit at a desk the whole day, drive home, eat and watch TV before rolling back into bed, then do the same the next day and the next day.

Forget about weight loss for a moment, and just look at the litany of the associated active health benefits. These include a lower risk of cardiovascular disease, stroke, hypertension, type 2 diabetes, osteoporosis, obesity, and cancer, and improved mood, sleep, trust, and sense of well-being. While many of the advantages of being active are driven by switching on our sirtuin genes, eating Sirtfoods should not be used as an excuse not to participate in the exercise. Rather we should appreciate how active the ideal complement to our consumption of Sirtfood is. It activates the sirtuin's full activation and all the benefits it brings, just as nature intends.

What we are talking about here is meeting the government guidelines of moderate physical activity for 150 minutes (2 hours and 30 minutes) a week. Strong work is the equivalent of a brisk walk. But that needn't be exclusive to it. Whichever sport or activity you enjoy is acceptable. Pleasure and exercise need not exclude one another! And its social aspect enriches even more team sports or community sports. It's also about daily things like taking the bike instead of the car or getting off the bus one stop earlier, or just parking farther away to increase the distance you have to walk about. Take the stairs and not the lift. Go outdoors and practice gardening. Play with your family in the park or get more out with your dog. These all count. All that has you up and going will activate your sirtuin genes frequently and at moderate strength, thus maximizing the benefits of the Sirtfood Diet. Engaging in physical exercise is giving your buck the full sirtuin bang while eating a diet rich in Sirtfood. What it takes is the equivalent of a brisk 30-minute stroll five days a week to achieve the benefit of physical activity.

Let's Wrap This Up!
- While the top twenty Sirtfoods should remain at the center of the plate, many other plants with sirtuin-activating properties should be included in our diets to make them diverse and varied.
- A diet rich in sirtfoods, complemented by the addition of animal products and fish, provides all the benefits of sirtuin activation and satisfies the need for other essential nutrients.
- While vegans and vegetarians can derive all the benefits from a Sirtfood diet, careful attention should be paid to those nutrients that may be lacking and appropriate food choices or supplements made.
- Sirtfood Diet followers are encouraged to engage in moderate activity for thirty minutes five times a week to reap the many benefits of well-being exercise and stimulate maximum activation of the sirtuin.

CHAPTER TEN: FREQUENTLY ASKED QUESTIONS AND ANSWERS

Should I do the Phase 1 exercise?

Daily exercise is one of the best things you can do for your wellbeing, and doing some moderate exercise can improve the diet's step 1 weight-loss and safety benefits. In general, we advise you to maintain your normal level of exercise and physical activity during the Sirtfood Diet's first seven days. However, we suggest staying in your normal comfort zone, as prolonged or excessively intense exercise can simply put too much stress on the body during this period. Check the body. There's no need to push yourself during Phase 1 for more exercise; instead, let the Sirtfoods do the hard work.

I'm Slim — Can I follow the diet still?

For anyone who is underweight, we do not recommend Phase 1 of the Sirtfood Diet. A reliable way of deciding whether you are underweight is to determine your body mass index or BMI. You can easily determine this by using one of the numerous online BMI calculators, as long as you know your height and weight. If your BMI is 18.5 or less, we do not recommend embarking on a diet phase 1. We should also recommend caution if your BMI is between 18.5 and 20, as following the diet can mean that your BMI falls below 18.5. While many people aspire to be super-skinny, the reality is that underweight can have a negative impact on many health aspects, contributing to a lower immune system, an increased risk of osteoporosis (weakening bones), and fertility issues. Though phase 1 of the diet is not recommended if you are underweight, we also promote the incorporation of plenty of Sirtfoods into a healthy way of eating so that all the health benefits of these foods can be reaped.

If you're slim but have a healthy range of BMI (20–25), however, there's absolutely nothing to stop you from getting started. A majority of the pilot trial participants had BMIs in the healthy range, but still lost impressive amounts of weight and got more toned. Importantly, many of them reported significantly improved energy, vitality, and appearance levels. Note that the Sirtfood Diet is about health promotion, as well as weight loss.

I'm Obese — is my Sirtfood diet, right?

Hey! Don't be put off by the fact that only a small minority of our pilot study participants were obese. This is because the pilot research was performed in a health and fitness club where participants are usually fitter and more aware of their wellbeing. Instead, be encouraged by the fact that the few who were obese had even better results than our participants who were healthy-weight. The thousands of people who tried the diet in the real world replicated those results. You should also stand to reap the greatest changes in your well-being, based on the research into sirtuin activation. Being obese increases the risk of many chronic health problems, yet these are the very illnesses against which Sirtfoods helps to protect.

I got my target weight and didn't want to lose anything more — do I stop eating syrups?

First of all, congratulations on your success in terms of weight loss! With Sirtfoods, you've had great success, but it doesn't stop now. Although we do not suggest more restrictions on calories, your diet will still provide enough Sirtfood. Many of our customers are now at their ideal body composition but continue to eat diets rich in Sirtfood. The best thing about Sirtfoods is they are a lifestyle. In terms of weight control, the best way to think of them is that they help get the body to the weight and shape it was meant to be. They work from here to maintain and keep you looking great and feeling great. Ultimately, this is the goal we wish for all followers of the Sirtfood Diet.

I finished Phase 2—Do I quit drinking Green Juice on the morning sirtfood now?

The green juice is our favorite way to start the day with a fantastic hit from Sirtfoods, so we endorse its long-term consumption. Our Sirtfood green juice has been carefully designed to include ingredients that provide a full spectrum of sirtuin-activating nutrients in potent dose-boosting fat-burning and wellness. We're all for variety, however, and while we recommend that you continue with a morning juice, we fully support anyone looking to experiment with various Sirtfood juice concoctions.

I'm taking medicine — is it OK to adopt the diet?

The Sirtfood Diet is suitable for most people, but due to its powerful effects on fat burning and health, it can alter the processes of certain diseases and the medication actions prescribed by your doctor. Similarly, other drugs are not appropriate in a state of fasting.

During the Sirtfood Diet trial, we assessed each individual's suitability before they embarked on the diet, particularly those taking medication. Obviously, we can't do that for you, so if you're suffering from a major health problem, taking prescribed medicines, or have other reasons to worry about getting into the diet, we recommend that you discuss it with your doctor first. The odds are it's going to be fine and profoundly beneficial for you, but testing is necessary.

If I am pregnant, can I follow the Diet?

If you are trying to conceive or are pregnant or breastfeeding, we do not recommend embarking on the Sirtfood Diet. It is a powerful diet for weight loss, which makes it inappropriate. Do not be put off eating plenty of Sirtfoods, however, as these are exceptionally healthy foods to be included as part of a balanced and varied pregnancy diet. Because of its alcohol content, you may want to avoid red wine and restrict caffeinated products such as coffee, green tea, and cocoa to not exceed 200 milligrams of caffeine per day during pregnancy (one mug of instant coffee usually contains about 100 milligrams of caffeine). Recommendations should not exceed four cups of green tea per day and should completely avoid matcha. Other than that, you are free to take advantage of having Sirtfoods included in your diet.

Are Sirtfoods Fit Children?

The Sirtfood Diet is a powerful diet for weight loss and not intended for kids. That doesn't mean that kids should miss out on the excellent health benefits offered by including more Sirtfoods in their overall diet, though. For children, a vast majority of Sirtfoods represent extremely healthy foods and help them achieve balanced and nutritious diets. Many of the recipes planned for the diet's Phase 2 have been developed with families in mind, including the taste buds of children. The likes of the Sirtfood pie, the chili con carne, and the Sirtfood bites are ideal child-friendly foods with a nutritional value higher than usual children's food offerings.

While most Sirtfoods are extremely healthy for children to eat, the green juice that is too concentrated in fat-burning sirtfoods is not recommended. We also advise against important caffeine sources, such as coffee and green tea. You will also need to be careful with chilies being included and may opt to keep things milder for kids.

Will I get a headache during Phase 1 or feel tired?

Phase 1 of the Sirtfood Diet provides powerful naturally occurring food compounds in amounts that most people wouldn't get into their normal diet, and some people can react as they adapt to this dramatic nutritional change. This may include symptoms such as mild headache or tiredness, although these effects are slight and short-lived in our experience.

Of course, if the symptoms are severe or give you cause for concern, we recommend that you seek medical advice promptly. Having said that, we have never seen anything other than occasional mild symptoms that rapidly resolve, and within a few days, most people find that they have a restored sense of vitality, vigor, and well-being.

Can I take additionals?

Unless your doctor or another health-care professional specifically prescribes for you, we do not recommend indiscriminate use of nutritional supplements. You will be ingesting from Sirtfoods a large and synergistic variety of natural plant compounds, and it is these that will do you good. You cannot replicate these benefits with nutritional supplements, and some nutritional supplements, such as antioxidants, may actually interfere with the beneficial effects of Sirtfoods, which is the last thing you want, especially if taken in high doses.

Whenever possible, we think that getting the nutrients you need from eating a balanced diet rich in Sirtfoods is much better than taking the nutrients in the form of a pill. Furthermore, because plant proteins are lower in leucine, the amino acid that enhances Sirtfoods' behavior, we have found that vegans can benefit from supplementing their diet with effective vegan protein powder. This applies in particular to those who practice high levels of exercise. This supplement should be taken off the Sirtfood green juice at a different time of day.

How often will I repeat phases 1 and 2?

You can repeat Phase 1 if you feel you need a weight-loss or a health boost. To ensure long-term negative effects of calorie restriction on your metabolism are not present, you should wait at least a month before repeating. But, in fact, we find that most people need to repeat it no more frequently than at most once every three months and continue to achieve amazing results. Instead, if you find that you've gone off track, need some fine-tuning, or want a bit more Sirtfood intensity, we recommend repeating as often as you like some or all of the Phase 2 days. Phase 2 is, after all, about establishing a lifelong way to eat. Note, the Sirtfood Diet's beauty is that it doesn't allow you to feel like you're constantly on a diet, but instead, it's the springboard to make meaningful lifestyle dietary changes that produce a lighter, leaner, healthier you.

Does the Sirtfood diet provide sufficient fiber?

Many Sirtfoods are, of course, fiber-rich. Onions, endive, and walnuts are notable sources, with buckwheat and Medjool dates really standing out, meaning the fiber department is not short of a Sirtfood-rich diet. Even during Phase 1, when food intake is reduced, most of us will still consume a quantity of fiber that we are used to, particularly if we select from the menu options the recipes that contain buckwheat, beans, and lentils. However, for others known to be susceptible to intestinal problems such as constipation without higher intakes of fiber, a suitable fiber supplement may be considered during Phase 1, especially Days 1 to 3, which should be discussed with your health care professional.

I read about superfoods — must I include them in my diet?

The first thing you need to say about the word superfood is that it's a marketing slogan and not a scientific concept at all. You don't need to worry about so-called superfoods because the Sirtfood Diet brings together the planet's healthiest foods into a revolutionary new way of eating. Just as relying on a simple vitamin pill to make us safe is a mistake, so relying on a single superfood to do the same is also a mistake. It is the entire diet, consisting of a wide spectrum of Sirtfoods and their vast array of natural compounds, acting in synergy, which is the true secret to achieving weight loss and lifelong health.

250 Sirtfood Diet Recipes

COPYRIGHT

All rights reserved. No part of this publication may be distributed, transmitted, or reproduced by any means or in any form, including photocopying, recording, or other electronic or mechanical methods, without the permission of the publisher, except in the case of brief quotations embodied in critical reviews and specific other noncommercial uses acceptable by copyright law.

Table of Contents

Green Juices Recipes 43

- Celery, Carrot & Orange Juice 44
- Orange & Kale Juice 44
- Apple, Carrot & Celery Juice 44
- Apple, Kale & Parsley Juice 44
- Apple, Cucumber & Celery Juice 44
- Apple & Celery Juice 44
- Kale & Apple Juice 45
- Kale & Celery Juice 45
- Apple, Orange & Broccoli Juice 45
- Kale, Carrot & Fruit Juice 45
- Kale, Celery, Apple & Orange Juice 45
- Kale, Celery & Pear Juice 46
- Green Fruit Juice 46
- Matcha, Apple & Greens Juice 46
- Parsley Green Juice 46
- Spinach & Apple Juice 46
- Parsley Creamy Juice 47
- Parsley Green Juice 47
- Mix Green Juice 47
- Rosemary Green Juice 47
- Cilantro & Lettuce Juice 47
- Cucumber Creamy Juice 48
- Kale & Kiwi Juice 48
- Broccoli Green Juice 48
- Berries Green Juice 48
- Fluffy Avocado Juice 49
- Broccoli Apple Juice 49
- Rocket Green Juice 49
- Swiss Chard Green Juice 49
- Kale Green Juice 50
- Arugula Leaves Juice 50
- Rocket Green Juice 50
- Lettuce Green Juice 50
- Broccoli Lime Juice 50
- Green Juice Recipe 51
- Healthy Green Juice With Lemon 51
- Green Juice For Beginners 51
- Tomato-Kale Gazpacho Smoothie 51
- My Favorite Green Juice 51
- Green Cleanse Smoothie 52
- Digestive Aid Green Juice 52
- Springtime Green Apple Juice 52
- Cilantro-Celery Juice Punch 52
- 4-Ingredient Fall Juice 52
- Best Green Juice Recipe 53
- Mix Green Juice 53
- Celery Green Juice 53
- Kale Green Juice 53
- Spinach & Apple Juice 53
- Cucumber Green Juice 54
- Creamy Spinach Juice 54

Breakfast Recipes 55

- Spinach Porridge 56
- Italian Spinach Tofu Omelet 56
- Tofu & Arugula Toast 56
- Breakfast Tofu Scramble 56
- Buckwheat & Walnuts Pancakes 57
- Breakfast Tofu Waffles 57
- Savory Buckwheat Porridge 57
- French Toast With Berries 57
- Buckwheat Crepe With Berries 58
- Kiwi & Apple Porridge 58
- Strawberry Smoothie Bowl 58
- Berries Pancakes 58
- Walnut Cream Parfait 59
- Chocolate Pancakes 59
- Tofu & Spinach Muffins 59
- Turmeric Tofu Toast 59
- Apple Bread Loaf 60
- Zucchini Tots 60
- Tofu & Berries Waffles 60
- Chocolate Pudding 60
- Cinnamon & Walnut Tea 61
- Apple Porridge 61
- Kale Omelet 61
- Tofu & Kale Toast 61
- Tofu Scramble 62
- Buckwheat Pancakes 62
- Waffle Sandwich 62
- Buckwheat Porridge 62
- Toast With Caramelized Apple 63
- Buckwheat Crepe With Apple 63
- Buckwheat & Apple Porridge 63
- Acai Berry Smoothie Bowl 63
- Walnuts Porridge 63
- Apple Pancakes 64
- Morning Parfait 64
- Spinach Muffins 64
- Chocolate Pancakes 64
- Buckwheat Bread Loaf 65
- Broccoli Muffins 65
- Buckwheat Waffles 65
- Eggless Pudding 65
- Turmeric Tea 66
- Buckwheat Granola 66
- Chocolate Granola 66
- Buckwheat Porridge With Berries 67
- Blueberry Pancakes 67
- Pumpkin Pancakes 67
- Matcha Pancakes 67
- Overnight Oat Pudding 68
- Zucchini And Chickpeas Frittata 68
- Walnuts Pudding With Oats 68

Homemade Walnut Bagels	69
Kale & Buckwheat Pancakes	69
Frutti & Nutty Breakfast Bowl	69
Pumpkin Porridge	69
Creamy Oat Porridge	69
Kale Muffins	70
Dates & Oats Bars	70
Chocolate Tea Latte	70
No Bake Brownies Bites	71
Kiwi Fruit Pudding	71
Baked French Toast With Berries	71
Kale & Chickpeas Omelet	71
Savory Zucchini Pancakes	71
Kale & Buckwheat Breakfast Bowl	72
Muesli Breakfast Bowl With Berries	72

Green Salads Recipes 73

Green Veggies Salad Bowl	74
Spinach & Lettuce Leaves Salad	74
Tofu Salad With Spinach	74
Tofu & Berries Salad	74
Pomegranate & Spinach Salad	74
Olives & Green Salad	75
Green Salad With Tofu	75
Arugula & Chicken Salad	75
Green Juicy Salad Bowl	75
Green Salad With Flaxseed	76
Green Salad With Spinach	76
Tabbouleh With Lime Dressing	76
Zucchini Olives And Beans Salad	76
Salmon Mushrooms And Lentils	77
Onion & Avocado Salad	77
Tuna & Veggies Salad	77
Watermelon & Raspberry Salad	77
Greek Salad With Olives	78
Salmon With Veggies	78
Lettuce Salad & Grilled Prawns	78

Main Meal Recipes 79

Creamy Spinach Curry	80
Broccoli Olives Pizza	80
Buffalo Broccoli Bites	80
Spinach Soup	80
Chili Tofu	81
Spicy Spinach Fillet	81
Broccoli Patties	81
Spinach & Tofu Pizza	82
Broccoli Flatbread Pizza	82
Turmeric Spinach Patties	82
Stir Fried Broccoli & Tofu	82
Wilted Spinach With Onion	83
Broccoli With Garlic Sauce	83
Hot & Sour Spinach	83
Spinach & Tofu Curry	83
Sardine Puttanesca Spaghetti	84
Tofu Power Bowls	84
Superfood Bibimbap With Crispy Tofu	85
Spicy Tofu Kale Wraps	85
Tofu Burritos	85
Asian Garlic Tofu	86
Tofu Burritos Recipe 2	86
Hot & Sour Soup	87
Tofu & Avocado Spring Rolls	87
Simple Tofu Quiche	87
Barbecued Waffle Iron Tofu	88
Cauliflower Mac 'N' Cheese	88
Beans & Broccolini	88
Chicken Stew	89
Baked Chicken With Salad	89
Lamb Chops With Salad	89
Flank Steak With Salad	90
Glazed Flank Steak	90
Salmon & Lentils	90
Salmon With Beans Salad	91
Tofu With Chickpeas & Kale	91
Beans & Veggie Salad	92
Buckwheat Noodles With Beef	92
Buckwheat Noodles With Shrimp	92
Chicken Breast With Asparagus	93
Slow Cooker Salmon & Walnut Soup	93
Salmon With Pesto & Beans	93
Mushrooms & Kale Stew	93
Grilled Crunchy Pepper	94
Stir Fried Shrimp & Kale	94
Stir Fry Shrimp & Broccoli	94
Chicken & Veggies Lunch Bowl	94
Lemon Fish Soup	95
Salmon & Potato Soup With Herbs	95
Sweet Corn Soup With Herbs	95
Prep Time 5 Min	95
Traditional Russian Cold Soup	96
Chicken Soup With Carrots	96
Chicken & Veggies Stew	96
Lentils Soup With Kale	96
Cauliflower & Broccoli Soup	97
Shrimp Soup With Cream	97
Kidney Beans & Tomato Soup	97
Walnut & Chicken Soup	97
Shrimp & Zucchini Stew	98
Beans & Veggies Soup	98
French Lentils Soup	98
Salmon & Beans Soup	98
Instant Pot Salmon Soup	98
Instant Pot Beans Soup	99
Detox Instant Veggies Stew	99
Instant Chicken & Veggies Stew	99
Instant Pot Kale Stew	100

Dessert & Snacks Recipes 101

Apple & Walnuts Cake	102
Baked Walnut Brownies	102
Coco & Walnuts Smoothie	102

- Walnut Cream Cake 102
- Walnuts Bits 102
- Walnuts Bites Muffins 103
- Buckwheat Cinnamon Buns 103
- Dates Brownies Bars 103
- Chocolate Pudding With Berries 103
- Dark Chocolate Cookies 104
- Homemade Walnut Milk 104
- Apple & Spinach Smoothie 104
- Homemade Walnut Cream 104
- Homemade Walnut Butter 104
- Cinnamon Chocolate Bites 105
- Walnut Ice-Cream 105
- Walnut Cream Smoothie 105
- Blueberries Smoothie 105
- Sirtfood Dates Bites 105
- Tofu & Blueberries Pie 106
- Easy Walnut Milk 106
- Healthy Berries Smoothie Bowl 106
- Kale & Walnut Dip 107
- Chocolate & Avocado Spread 107
- Chicken Snacks 107
- Garlic & Cucumber Dip 107
- Chocolate Smoothie Jar 107
- Beet Root & Kale Hummus 107
- Walnut Dip 108
- Turmeric & Olives Hummus 108
- Chocolate Whipped Cream 108
- Creamy Avocado Sauce 108
- Healthy Matcha Tea Smoothie 108
- Spicy Shrimp Wrap 108

Green Juices Recipes

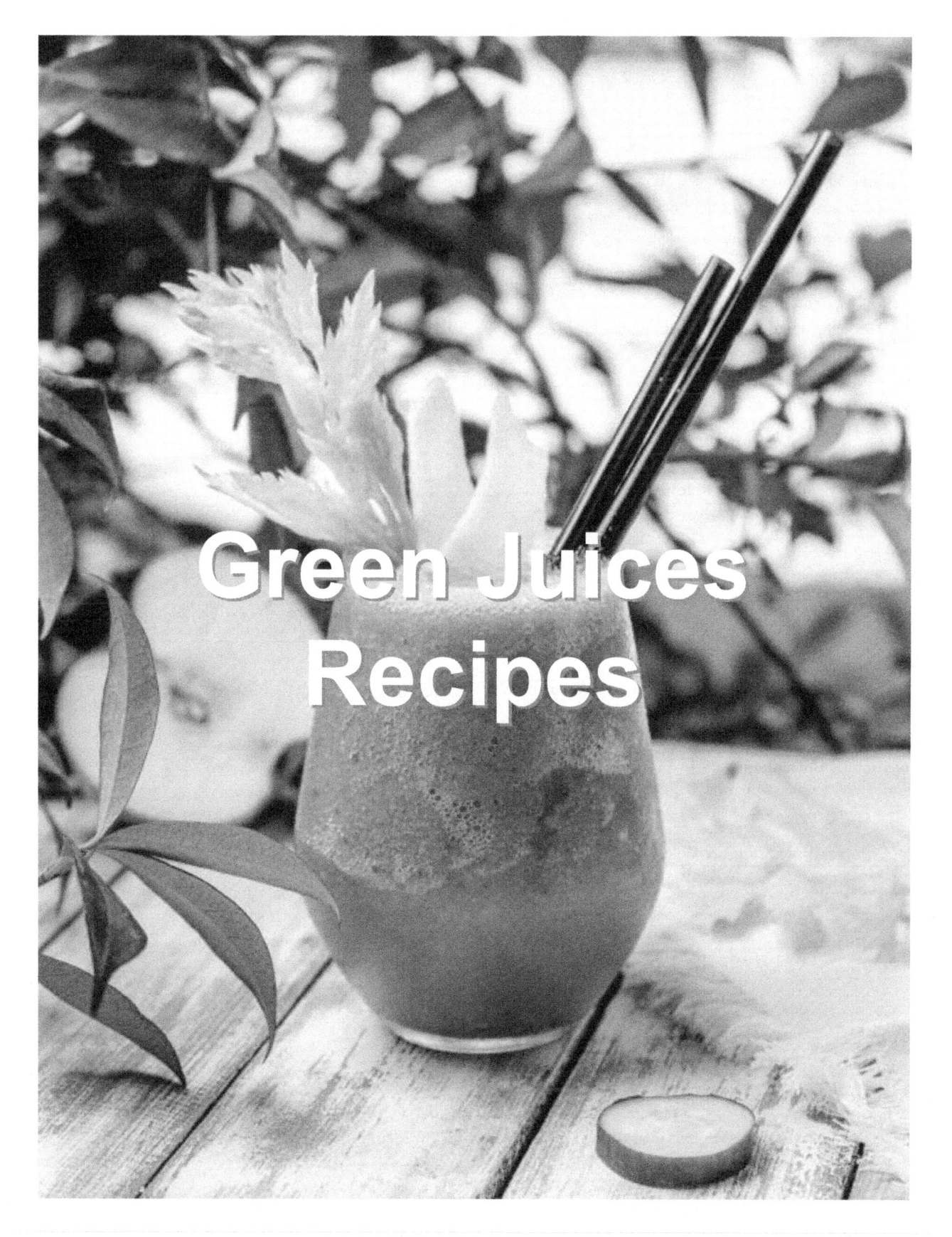

Celery, Carrot & Orange Juice

Prep Time 10 min

Servings 2

Ingredients:
- 4 celery stalks with leaves
- 3 medium carrots, peeled and chopped
- 2 oranges, peeled and sectioned
- 1 tablespoon fresh ginger, peeled

Directions:
1. Place all ingredients in a high-powered blender and pulse until well combined.
2. Through a fine mesh strainer, strain the juice and transfer it into two glasses.
3. Serve immediately.

Nutritional information:
Calories Per Servings, 181 kcal, 1.72 g Fat, 39.64 g Total Carbs, 10.41 g Protein, 12.2 g Fiber

Orange & Kale Juice

Prep Time 10 min

Servings 2

Ingredients:
- 4 large oranges, peeled and sectioned
- 2 bunches fresh kale

Directions:
1. Put all ingredients in a juicer and extract the juice according to the manufacturer's instructions.
2. Pour into two glasses and serve immediately.

Nutritional information:
Calories Per Servings, 181 kcal, 0.4 g Fat, 57 g Total Carbs, 10.41 g Protein, 7 g Fiber

Apple, Carrot & Celery Juice

Prep Time 10 min

Servings 2

Ingredients:
- 5 carrots, peeled and chopped
- 1 large apple, cored and chopped
- 2 celery stalks
- 1 (½-inch) piece fresh ginger, peeled and chopped
- ½ of lemon

Directions:
1. Put all ingredients in a juicer and extract the juice according to the manufacturer's instructions.
2. Pour into two glasses and serve immediately.

Nutritional information:
Calories Per Servings, 126 kcal, 0.3 g Fat, 31 g Total Carbs, 1 g Protein, 6 g Fiber

Apple, Kale & Parsley Juice

Prep Time 10 min

Servings 2

Ingredients:
- 2 large green apples, cored and sliced
- 4 cups fresh kale leaves
- 4 tablespoons fresh parsley leaves
- 1 tablespoon fresh ginger, peeled
- 1 lemon, peeled
- ½ cup filtered water
- Pinch of salt

Directions:
1. Place all ingredients in a high-powered blender and pulse until well combined.
2. Through a fine mesh strainer, strain the juice and transfer it into two glasses.
3. Serve immediately.

Nutritional information:
Calories Per Servings, 197 kcal, 0.7 g Fat, 48 g Total Carbs, 5 g Protein, 8 g Fiber

Apple, Cucumber & Celery Juice

Prep Time 10 min

Servings 2

Ingredients:
- 3 large apples, cored and sliced
- 2 large cucumbers, sliced
- 4 celery stalks
- 1 (1-inch) piece fresh ginger, peeled
- 1 lemon, peeled

Directions:
1. Put all ingredients in a juicer and extract the juice according to the manufacturer's instructions.
2. Pour into two glasses and serve immediately.

Nutritional information:
Calories Per Servings, 230 kcal, 1 g Fat, 59 g Total Carbs, 3 g Protein, 10 g Fiber

Apple & Celery Juice

Prep Time 10 min

Servings 2

Ingredients:
- 4 large green apples, cored and sliced
- 4 celery stalks

- 1 lemon, peeled

Directions:
1. Put all ingredients in a juicer and extract the juice according to the manufacturer's instructions.
2. Pour into two glasses and serve immediately.

Nutritional information:
Calories Per Servings, 240 kcal, 0.9 g Fat, 63 g Total Carbs, 1 g Protein, 11 g Fiber

Kale & Apple Juice

Prep Time 10 min

Servings 2

Ingredients:
- 3 large green apples, cored and sliced
- 4 cups fresh kale leaves
- 2 tablespoons fresh lemon juice
- ½ cup filtered water

Directions:
1. Put all ingredients in a juicer and extract the juice according to the manufacturer's instructions.
2. Pour into two glasses and serve immediately.

Nutritional information:
Calories Per Servings, 244 kcal, 0.7 g Fat, 60 g Total Carbs, 5 g Protein, 10 g Fiber

Kale & Celery Juice

Prep Time 10 min

Servings 2

Ingredients:
- 4 celery stalks
- 5 cups fresh kale leaves
- 1 (½-inch) piece fresh ginger, peeled
- 1 lime, halved

Directions:
1. Put all ingredients in a juicer and extract the juice according to the manufacturer's instructions.
2. Pour into two glasses and serve immediately.

Nutritional information:
Calories Per Servings, 91 kcal, 0.1 g Fat, 19 g Total Carbs, 5 g Protein, 3 g Fiber

Apple, Orange & Broccoli Juice

Prep Time 10 min

Servings 2

Ingredients:
- 2 broccoli stalks, chopped
- 2 large green apples, cored and sliced
- 3 large oranges, peeled and sectioned
- 4 tablespoons fresh parsley

Directions:
1. Put all ingredients in a juicer and extract the juice according to the manufacturer's instructions.
2. Pour into two glasses and serve immediately.

Nutritional information:
Calories Per Servings, 254 kcal, 0.8 g Fat, 64 g Total Carbs, 3 g Protein, 12 g Fiber

Kale, Carrot & Fruit Juice

Prep Time 10 min

Servings 2

Ingredients:
- 3 cups fresh kale
- 2 large apples, cored and sliced
- 2 medium carrots, peeled and chopped
- 2 medium grapefruit, peeled and sectioned
- 1 teaspoon fresh lemon juice

Directions:
1. Put all ingredients in a juicer and extract the juice according to the manufacturer's instructions.
2. Pour into two glasses and serve immediately.

Nutritional information:
Calories Per Servings, 232 kcal, 0 g Fat, 57g Total Carbs, 4 g Protein, 9 g Fiber

Kale, Celery, Apple & Orange Juice

Prep Time 10 min

Servings 2

Ingredients:
- 3 cups fresh kale, chopped
- 2 large celery stalks, chopped
- 2 large green apples, cored and sliced
- 1 large orange, peeled and sectioned
- 1 tablespoon fresh lime juice
- 1 tablespoon fresh lemon juice

Directions:
1. Put all ingredients in a juicer and extract the juice according to the manufacturer's instructions.
2. Pour into two glasses and serve immediately.

Nutritional information:
Calories Per Servings, 214 kcal, 0.1 g Fat, 52 g Total Carbs, 4 g Protein, 9 g Fiber

Kale, Celery & Pear Juice

Prep Time 10 min

Servings 2

Ingredients:
- 6 pears, cored and chopped
- 3 celery stalks
- 3 cups fresh kale
- 2 tablespoons fresh parsley

Directions:
1. Put all ingredients in a juicer and extract the juice according to the manufacturer's instructions.
2. Pour into two glasses and serve immediately.

Nutritional information:
Calories Per Servings, 209 kcal, 0.9g Fat, 50 g Total Carbs, 5 g Protein, 15 g Fiber

Green Fruit Juice

Prep Time 10 min

Servings 2

Ingredients:
- 3 large kiwis, peeled and chopped
- 2 large green apples, cored and sliced
- 2 cups seedless green grapes
- 2 teaspoons fresh lime juice

Directions:
1. Put all ingredients in a juicer and extract the juice according to the manufacturer's instructions.
2. Pour into two glasses and serve immediately.

Nutritional information:
Calories Per Servings, 265 kcal, 0.6g Fat, 68 g Total Carbs, 1 g Protein, 9 g Fiber

Matcha, Apple &Greens Juice

Prep Time 10 min

Servings 2

Ingredients:
- 5 ounces fresh kale
- 2 ounces fresh arugula
- ¼ cup fresh parsley
- 4 celery stalks
- 1 green apple, cored and chopped
- 1 (1-inch) piece fresh ginger, peeled
- 1 lemon, peeled
- ½ teaspoon matcha green tea

Directions:
1. Put all ingredients in a juicer and extract the juice according to the manufacturer's instructions.
2. Pour into two glasses and serve immediately.

Nutritional information:
Calories Per Servings, 113 kcal, 0.6 g Fat, 26 g Total Carbs, 3 g Protein, 5 g Fiber

Parsley Green Juice

Prep Time 10 min

Servings 1

Ingredients:
- 1 bunch parsley
- 1 kiwi fruit
- 1 cucumber
- 1 apple
- half a lemon, juiced
- 1 tsp. matcha green tea

Directions:
1. Put parsley, apple, cucumber, and kiwi fruit in an electric juicer and extract the juice.
2. Pour the juice into a glass and mix matcha, lemon juice with a fork.
3. Once the matcha tea powder is mixed in juice add some water.
4. Pour some ice on top.
5. Enjoy!

Nutritional information:
Calories Per Servings, 181 kcal, 1.72 g Fat, 39.64 g Total Carbs, 10.41 g Protein, 12.2 g Fiber

Spinach & Apple Juice

Prep Time 10 min

Servings 1

Ingredients:
- 1 bunch baby spinach
- 1 apple
- ¼ cup mixed berries
- 1/8 tsp. ginger
- half a lemon, juiced
- 1 tsp. matcha green tea

Directions:
1. Put spinach, apple, and berries in an electric juicer and extract the juice.
2. Pour the juice into a glass and mix matcha, lemon juice with a fork.
3. Once the matcha tea powder is mixed in juice add some water.
4. Pour some ice on top.
5. Enjoy!

Nutritional information:
Calories Per Servings, 121 kcal, 0.49 g Fat, 32.2 g Total Carbs, 0.85 g Protein, 5.3 g Fiber

Parsley Creamy Juice

Prep Time 10 min

Servings 1

Ingredients:
- 1 bunch parsley
- 1 green apple
- 1 cup broccoli
- 1/8 tsp ginger
- ¼ cup walnut milk
- half a lemon, juiced
- 1 tsp. matcha green tea

Directions:
1. Put parsley, apple, broccoli, and ginger in an electric juicer and extract the juice.
2. Pour the juice into a glass and mix matcha, lemon juice with a fork.
3. Once the matcha tea powder is mixed in juice add some water and milk
4. Pour some ice on top.
5. Enjoy!

Nutritional information:
Calories Per Servings, 187 kcal, 1.89 g Fat, 40.33 g Total Carbs, 11.56 g Protein, 13 g Fiber

Parsley Green Juice

Prep Time 10 min

Servings 1

Ingredients:
- 1 bunch parsley leaves
- 2 stalk celery
- 1 apple
- half a lemon, juiced
- 1 tsp. matcha green tea

Directions:
1. Put parsley, apple, and celery in an electric juicer and extract the juice.
2. Pour the juice into a glass and mix matcha, lemon juice with a fork.
3. Once the matcha tea powder is mixed in juice add some water.
4. Pour some ice on top.
5. Enjoy!

Nutritional information:
Calories Per Servings, 118 kcal, 0.55 g Fat, 3o.07 g Total Carbs, 1.33 g Protein, 6.2 g Fiber

Mix Green Juice

Prep Time 10 min

Servings 1

Ingredients:
- 1 bunch spinach leaves
- 1 apple
- 1 cucumber
- half a lemon, juiced
- 1 tsp. matcha green tea

Directions:
1. Put spinach, apple, cucumber, and kiwi fruit in an electric juicer and extract the juice.
2. Pour the juice into a glass and mix matcha, lemon juice with a fork.
3. Once the matcha tea powder is mixed in juice add some water.
4. Pour some ice on top.
5. Enjoy!

Nutritional information:
Calories Per Servings, 146 kcal, 1.16 g Fat, 33.93 g Total Carbs, 3.53 g Protein, 7.8 g Fiber

Rosemary Green Juice

Prep Time 10 min

Servings 1

Ingredients:
- 2 bunch baby spinach
- 1 cup chopped rosemary
- 1 apple
- 1 cucumber
- ¼ cup walnut milk
- half a lemon, juiced
- 1 tsp. matcha green tea

Directions:
1. Put spinach, rosemary, apple, cucumber in an electric juicer and extract the juice.
2. Pour the juice into a glass and mix matcha, lemon juice with a fork.
3. Once the matcha tea powder is mixed in juice add some water and walnut milk.
4. Pour some ice on top.
5. Enjoy!

Nutritional information:
Calories Per Servings, 171 kcal, 1.67 g Fat, 39.53 g Total Carbs, 6.54 g Protein, 9.8 g Fiber

Cilantro & Lettuce Juice

Prep Time 10 min

Servings 1

Ingredients:
- 1 bunch cilantro leaves
- 4-5 lettuce leaves
- 1 apple
- half a lemon, juiced
- 1 tsp. matcha green tea

Directions:
1. Put cilantro, apple, and lettuce in an electric juicer and extract the juice.
2. Pour the juice into a glass and mix matcha, lemon juice with a fork.
3. Once the matcha tea powder is mixed in juice add some water.
4. Pour some ice on top.
5. Enjoy!

Nutritional information:
Calories Per Servings, 178 kcal, 1.69 g Fat, 39.13 g Total Carbs, 10.29 g Protein, 11.9 g Fiber

Cucumber Creamy Juice

Prep Time 10 min

Servings 19

Ingredients:
- 2 cucumbers
- 1 green apple
- ¼ cup walnut milk
- half a lemon, juiced
- 1 tsp. matcha green tea

Directions:
1. Put cucumber, apple in an electric juicer and extract the juice.
2. Pour the juice into a glass and mix matcha, lemon juice with a fork.
3. Once the matcha tea powder is mixed in juice add some water and walnut milk.
4. Pour some ice on top.
5. Enjoy!

Nutritional information:
Calories Per Servings, 124 kcal, 0.69 g Fat, 31.13 g Total Carbs, 1.75 g Protein, 5.8 g Fiber

Kale & Kiwi Juice

Prep Time 10 min

Servings 1

Ingredients:
- 1 bunch kale
- ½ cup soy milk
- 1 kiwi fruit
- half a medium green apple
- half a lemon, juiced
- 1 tsp. matcha green tea

Directions:
1. Put kale and kiwi fruit in an electric juicer and extract the juice.
2. Pour the juice into a glass and mix matcha, lemon juice with a fork.
3. Once the matcha tea powder is mixed in juice add some water and soy milk.
4. Pour some ice on top.
5. Enjoy!

Nutritional information:
Calories Per Servings, 185 kcal, 3.35 g Fat, 32.68 g Total Carbs, 13.28 g Protein, 10 g Fiber

Broccoli Green Juice

Prep Time 10 min

Servings 1

Ingredients:
- 1 head broccoli
- 1 bunch spinach leaves
- 1 apple
- half a lemon, juiced
- 1 tsp. matcha green tea

Directions:
1. Put broccoli, spinach, apple in an electric juicer and extract the juice.
2. Pour the juice into a glass and mix matcha, lemon juice with a fork.
3. Once the matcha tea powder is mixed in juice add some water.
4. Pour some ice on top.
5. Enjoy!

Nutritional information:
Calories Per Servings, 124 kcal, 0.87 g Fat, 31.9 g Total Carbs, 2.47 g Protein, 6.7 g Fiber

Berries Green Juice

Prep Time 10 min

Servings 1

Ingredients:
- 1 bunch mint leaves
- 1 apple
- large stalks green celery, including leaves
- 1 cup mixed berries
- half a lemon, juiced
- 1 tsp. matcha green tea

Directions:
1. Put mint leaves, apple, celery, and berries in an electric juicer and extract the juice.

2. Pour the juice into a glass and mix matcha, lemon juice with a fork.
3. Once the matcha tea powder is mixed in juice add some water.
4. Pour some ice on top.
5. Enjoy!

Nutritional information:
Calories Per Servings, 181 kcal, 1.72 g Fat, 39.64 g Total Carbs, 10.41 g Protein, 12.2 g Fiber

Fluffy Avocado Juice

Prep Time 10 min

Servings 1

Ingredients:
- 1 head broccoli
- 1 apple
- ¼ cup avocado
- 1/8 tsp. ginger
- half a lemon, juiced
- 1 tsp. matcha green tea

Directions:
1. Put broccoli, apple, avocado, and ginger in an electric juicer and extract the juice.
2. Pour the juice into a glass and mix matcha, lemon juice with a fork.
3. Once the matcha tea powder is mixed in juice add some water.
4. Pour some ice on top.
5. Enjoy!

Nutritional information:
Calories Per Servings, 121 kcal, 0.49 g Fat, 32.2 g Total Carbs, 0.85 g Protein, 5.3 g Fiber

Broccoli Apple Juice

Prep Time 10 min

Servings 1

Ingredients:
- 1 bunch spinach
- 1 apple
- 1 cup broccoli
- 1/8 tsp ginger
- half a lemon, juiced
- 1 tsp. matcha green tea

Directions:
1. Put spinach, apple, broccoli, and ginger in an electric juicer and extract the juice.
2. Pour the juice into a glass and mix matcha, lemon juice with a fork.
3. Once the matcha tea powder is mixed in juice add some water.

4. Pour some ice on top.
5. Enjoy!

Nutritional information:
Calories Per Servings, 187 kcal, 1.89 g Fat, 40.33 g Total Carbs, 11.56 g Protein, 13 g Fiber
\

Rocket Green Juice

Prep Time 10 min

Servings 1

Ingredients:
- 1 rocket leaves
- 1 apple
- 1 cucumber
- half a lemon, juiced
- 1 tsp. matcha green tea

Directions:
1. Put rocket leaves, apples, and cucumber in an electric juicer and extract the juice.
2. Pour the juice into a glass and mix matcha and lemon juice with a fork.
3. Once the matcha tea powder is mixed in juice, add some water.
4. Pour some ice on top.
5. Enjoy!

Nutritional information:
Calories Per Servings, 146 kcal, 1.16 g Fat, 33.93 g Total Carbs, 3.53 g Protein, 7.8 g Fiber

Swiss Chard Green Juice

Prep Time 10 min

Servings 1

Ingredients:
- 1 bunch swiss chard leaves
- 1 apple
- half a lemon, juiced
- 1 tsp. matcha green tea

Directions:
1. Put Swiss chard leaves, apple in an electric juicer and extract the juice.
2. Pour the juice into a glass and mix matcha, lemon juice with a fork.
3. Once the matcha tea powder is mixed in juice add some water.
4. Pour some ice on top.
5. Enjoy!

Nutritional information:
Calories Per Servings, 118 kcal, 0.55 g Fat, 30.07 g Total Carbs, 1.33 g Protein, 6.2 g Fiber

Kale Green Juice

Prep Time 10 min

Servings 1

Ingredients:
- 2 bunch kale
- 1 apple
- 2 stalk celery with leaves
- half a lemon, juiced
- 1 tsp. matcha green tea

Directions:
1. Put kale, apple, celery in electric juice and extract the juice.
2. Pour the juice into a glass and mix in matcha and lemon juice with a fork.
3. Once the matcha tea powder is mixed in juice add some water.
4. Pour some ice on top.
5. Enjoy!

Nutritional information:
Calories Per Servings, 171 kcal, 1.67 g Fat, 39.53 g Total Carbs, 6.54 g Protein, 9.8 g Fiber

Arugula leaves Juice

Prep Time 10 min

Servings 1

Ingredients:
- 1 bunch arugula leaves
- 1 apple
- half a lemon, juiced
- 1 tsp. matcha green tea

Directions:
1. Put arugula leaves, apple, in electric juice and extract the juice.
2. Pour the juice into a glass and mix matcha, lemon juice with a fork.
3. Once the matcha tea powder is mixed in juice add some water.
4. Pour some ice on top.
5. Enjoy!

Nutritional information:
Calories Per Servings, 178 kcal, 1.69 g Fat, 39.13 g Total Carbs, 10.29 g Protein, 11.9 g Fiber

Rocket Green Juice

Prep Time 10 min

Servings 1

Ingredients:
- 1 cucumber
- 1 green apple
- half a lemon, juiced
- 1 tsp. matcha green tea

Directions:
1. Put parsley, apple, cucumber, and kiwi fruit in an electric juicer and extract the juice.
2. Pour the juice into a glass and mix matcha, lemon juice with a fork.
3. Once the matcha tea powder is mixed in juice add some water.
4. Pour some ice on top.
5. Enjoy!

Nutritional information:
Calories Per Servings, 124 kcal, 0.69 g Fat, 31.13 g Total Carbs, 1.75 g Protein, 5.8 g Fiber

Lettuce Green Juice

Prep Time 10 min

Servings 1

Ingredients:
- 1 bunch lettuce leaves
- ½ cup soy milk
- half a medium green apple
- 1 stalk celery
- half a lemon, juiced
- 1 tsp. matcha green tea

Directions:
1. Put lettuce leaves, apple, and celery in an electric juicer and extract the juice.
2. Pour the juice into a glass and mix matcha, lemon juice with a fork.
3. Once the matcha tea powder is mixed in juice add some water and soy milk.
4. Pour some ice on top.
5. Enjoy!

Nutritional information:
Calories Per Servings, 185 kcal, 3.35 g Fat, 32.68 g Total Carbs, 13.28 g Protein, 10 g Fiber

Broccoli Lime Juice

Prep Time 10 min

Servings 1

Ingredients:
- 1 cup broccoli
- 1 apple
- ¼ cup lime juice
- 1 tsp. matcha green tea

Directions:
1. Put broccoli in an electric juicer and extract the juice.

2. Pour the juice into a glass and mix matcha, lime juice with a fork.
3. Once the matcha tea powder is mixed in juice add some water.
4. Pour some ice on top.
5. Enjoy!

Nutritional information:
Calories Per Servings, 124 kcal, 0.87 g Fat, 31.9 g Total Carbs, 2.47 g Protein, 6.7 g Fiber

Green Juice Recipe

Prep Time 15 min

Servings 2

Ingredients:
- 1 bunch curly kale roughly chopped
- 1 large lemon peeled and quartered
- 1-inch ginger peeled
- 1 large cucumber cut into long strips
- 2 large granny smith apples cored and sliced
- 4 whole celery stalks

Directions:
1. Put broccoli in an electric juicer and extract the juice.
2. Pour the juice into a glass and mix matcha, lime juice with a fork.
3. Once the matcha tea powder is mixed in juice add some water.
4. Pour some ice on top.
5. Enjoy!

Nutritional information:
Calories Per Servings, 124 kcal, 0.87 g Fat, 31.9 g Total Carbs, 2.47 g Protein, 6.7 g Fiber

Healthy Green Juice with Lemon

Prep Time 10 min

Servings 1

Ingredients:
- 1 bunch of kale
- 1 head romaine lettuce
- 1 medium carrot optional
- 5 celery stalks
- 1 medium cucumber
- 1 green apple
- 2 lemons
- 1" piece of fresh ginger

Directions:
1. Wash all your Ingredients.
2. Juice Ingredients according to your juicer's instruction manual. If you don't have a juicer, you can use the blender method (see above).
3. Sip slowly and enjoy

Nutritional information:
Calories Per Servings, 124 kcal, 0.87 g Fat, 31.9 g Total Carbs, 2.47 g Protein, 6.7 g Fiber

Green Juice for Beginners

Prep Time 10 min

Servings 1

Ingredients:
- 2 pears
- 2 handfuls of fresh spinach (about 1.5 oz or 40 g)
- 1 stalk of celery
- 0.5-inch piece of ginger root (about 1cm)
- 1/4 fennel bulb (or 2 stalks of celery)

Directions:
1. Wash and chop all the ingredients. You don't need to peel the pears or the ginger root, although if they're not organic you should.
2. Put everything through the juicer.
3. Our juicer has a strainer, so we don't strain the juice, but if your juicer hasn't one, maybe you want to strainer your juice to get a better texture, it's up to you.

Nutritional information:
Calories Per Servings, 124 kcal, 0.87 g Fat, 31.9 g Total Carbs, 2.47 g Protein, 6.7 g Fiber

Tomato-Kale Gazpacho Smoothie

Prep Time 10 min

Servings 1

Ingredients:
- 1/4 c. water
- 2 tbsp. lime juice
- 1/2 c. plain Greek yogurt
- 1/4 tsp. ground cumin
- 2 large kale leaves, stems removed
- 1 c. fresh or canned diced tomatoes
- 1 small carrot, chopped
- 1 small cucumber, chopped
- 1/2 rib celery, chopped
- 1/2 c. ice

Directions:
1. Add hot sauce to taste and blend until smooth. Divide between 2 glasses.

Nutritional information:
Calories Per Servings, 124 kcal, 0.87 g Fat, 31.9 g Total Carbs, 2.47 g Protein, 6.7 g Fiber

My Favorite Green Juice

Prep Time 10 min

Servings 1

Ingredients:
- 1 head of romaine lettuce
- 2 large kale leaves
- Handful of fresh parsley
- 1 large Granny Smith apple, chopped
- 2 lemons, peeled
- 1 cup broccoli

Directions:
1. Put all ingredients in a juicer and extract the juice.
2. Pour the juice into a glass.
3. Pour some ice on top.
4. Enjoy!

Nutritional information:
Calories Per Servings, 124 kcal, 0.87 g Fat, 31.9 g Total Carbs, 2.47 g Protein, 6.7 g Fiber

Green Cleanse Smoothie

Prep Time 10 min

Servings 1

Ingredients:
- 1 cup chopped pineapple
- 1 small handful of spinach, chopped
- 1 kiwi fruit, peeled and chopped
- 1 cup of coconut water

Directions:
1. Put all ingredients in a juicer and extract the juice.
2. Pour the juice into a glass.
3. Pour some ice on top.
4. Enjoy!

Nutritional information:
Calories Per Servings, 124 kcal, 0.87 g Fat, 31.9 g Total Carbs, 2.47 g Protein, 6.7 g Fiber

Digestive Aid Green Juice

Prep Time 10 min

Servings 1

Ingredients:
- 1 celery stick
- 2 handfuls of fresh kale
- 1/4 fennel**
- 1/2-inch piece of ginger root (about 1 cm)
- 2 pears

Directions:
1. Put all ingredients in a juicer and extract the juice.
2. Pour the juice into a glass.
3. Pour some ice on top.
4. Enjoy!

Nutritional information:
Calories Per Servings, 124 kcal, 0.87 g Fat, 31.9 g Total Carbs, 2.47 g Protein, 6.7 g Fiber

Springtime Green Apple Juice

Prep Time 10 min

Servings 1

Ingredients:
- 1 green apple, cored
- 4 celery stalks
- 1/2 medium cucumber
- 1/2-inch fresh ginger

Directions:
1. Put all ingredients in a juicer and extract the juice.
2. Pour the juice into a glass.
3. Pour some ice on top.
4. Enjoy!

Nutritional information:
Calories Per Servings, 124 kcal, 0.87 g Fat, 31.9 g Total Carbs, 2.47 g Protein, 6.7 g Fiber

Cilantro-Celery Juice Punch

Prep Time 10 min

Servings 1

Ingredients:
- 1-piece fresh ginger (about 1/2 ounce)
- 1 bunch cilantro (about 4 ounces)
- 1 Granny Smith apple
- 8 rib(s) celery
- 2 tsp. lemon juice

Directions:
1. In an electric juicer, juice the ginger, cilantro, apple, and celery.
2. Stir in the lemon juice and serve right away.

Nutritional information:
Calories Per Servings, 124 kcal, 0.87 g Fat, 31.9 g Total Carbs, 2.47 g Protein, 6.7 g Fiber

4-Ingredient Fall Juice

Prep Time 10 min

Servings 1

Ingredients:
- 6 apples
- 2 oranges
- 4 cups Swiss chard (145 g)
- 2 celery sticks

Directions:
1. Wash all the Ingredients.

2. Peel the oranges.
3. Chop the fruits and veggies.
4. Put everything through the juicer.
5. Strain the juice for a better texture (optional)

Nutritional information:
Calories Per Servings, 124 kcal, 0.87 g Fat, 31.9 g Total Carbs, 2.47 g Protein, 6.7 g Fiber

BEST GREEN JUICE RECIPE

Prep Time 10 min

Servings 1

Ingredients:
- 1 cucumber, sliced
- 3 stalks celery, sliced
- 3 leaves kale, removed from stem
- 1 cup spinach, baby leaves, loosely packed
- 1-piece fresh ginger, approx. 1–2-inch chunk
- 2 tablespoons lime juice
- 2 apples, cored and sliced

Directions:
1. Put all ingredients in a juicer and extract the juice.
2. Pour the juice into a glass.
3. Pour some ice on top.
4. Enjoy!

Mix Green Juice

Prep Time 10 min

Servings 1

Ingredients:
- 1 bunch parsley
- 1 apple
- 1 cucumber
- half a lemon, juiced
- 1 tsp. matcha green tea

Directions:
1. Extract the juice of parsley apple and cucumber.
2. Pour a Half juice into a glass, then add the matcha, lemon juice and mix well with a fork.
3. Once the matcha is dissolved add the
4. remainder of the juice.
5. Mix well.
6. Pour some water on top.
7. Enjoy!

Nutritional information:
Calories Per Servings, 146 kcal, 1.16 g Fat, 33.93 g Total Carbs, 3.53 g Protein, 7.8 g Fiber

Celery Green Juice

Prep Time 10 min

Servings 1

Ingredients:
- 5 -8 stalks celery with leaves
- 1 apple
- half a lemon, juiced
- 1 tsp. matcha green tea

Directions:
1. Extract the juice of celery and apple.
2. Pour a Half juice into a glass, then add the matcha, lemon juice and mix well with a fork.
3. Once the matcha is dissolved add the
4. remainder of the juice.
5. Mix well.
6. Pour some water on top.
7. Enjoy!

Nutritional information:
Calories Per Servings, 118 kcal, 0.55 g Fat, 30.07 g Total Carbs, 1.33 g Protein, 6.2 g Fiber

Kale Green Juice

Prep Time 10 min

Servings 1

Ingredients:
- 2 bunch kale
- 1 apple
- 2 stalk celery with leaves
- half a lemon, juiced
- 1 tsp. matcha green tea

Directions:
1. Extract the juice of kale, apple, and celery.
2. Pour a Half juice into a glass, then add the matcha, lemon juice and mix well with a fork.
3. Once the matcha is dissolved add the
4. remainder of the juice.
5. Mix well.
6. Pour some water on top.
7. Enjoy!

Nutritional information:
Calories Per Servings, 171 kcal, 1.67 g Fat, 39.53 g Total Carbs, 6.54 g Protein, 9.8 g Fiber

Spinach & Apple Juice

Prep Time 10 min

Servings 1

Ingredients:
- 1 bunch baby spinach
- 1 apple

- half a lemon, juiced
- 1 tsp. matcha green tea

Directions:
1. Extract the juice of spinach and apple.
2. Pour a Half juice into a glass, then add the matcha, lemon juice and mix well with a fork.
3. Once the matcha is dissolved add the
4. remainder of the juice.
5. Mix well.
6. Pour some water on top.
7. Enjoy!

Nutritional information:
Calories Per Servings, 178 kcal, 1.69 g Fat, 39.13 g Total Carbs, 10.29 g Protein, 11.9 g Fiber

Cucumber Green Juice

Prep Time 10 min

Servings 1

Ingredients:
- 1 cucumber
- 1 green apple
- half a lemon, juiced
- 1 tsp. matcha green tea

Directions:
1. Extract the juice of cucumber and apple.
2. Pour a Half juice into a glass, then add the matcha, lemon juice and mix well with a fork.
3. Once the matcha is dissolved add the
4. remainder of the juice.
5. Mix well.
6. Pour some water on top.
7. Enjoy!

Nutritional information:
Calories Per Servings, 124 kcal, 0.69 g Fat, 31.13 g Total Carbs, 1.75 g Protein, 5.8 g Fiber

Creamy Spinach Juice

Prep Time 10 min

Servings 1

Ingredients:
- 1 bunch spinach
- ½ cup soy milk
- half a medium green apple
- half a lemon, juiced
- 1 tsp. matcha green tea

Directions:
1. Extract the juice of spinach and apple.
2. Pour a Half juice into a glass, then add the matcha, lemon juice and mix well with a fork.
3. Once the matcha is dissolved add the
4. remainder of the juice.
5. Mix well.
6. Pour some water on top.
7. Enjoy!

Nutritional information:
Calories Per Servings, 185 kcal, 3.35 g Fat, 32.68 g Total Carbs, 13.28 g Protein, 10 g Fiber

Breakfast Recipes

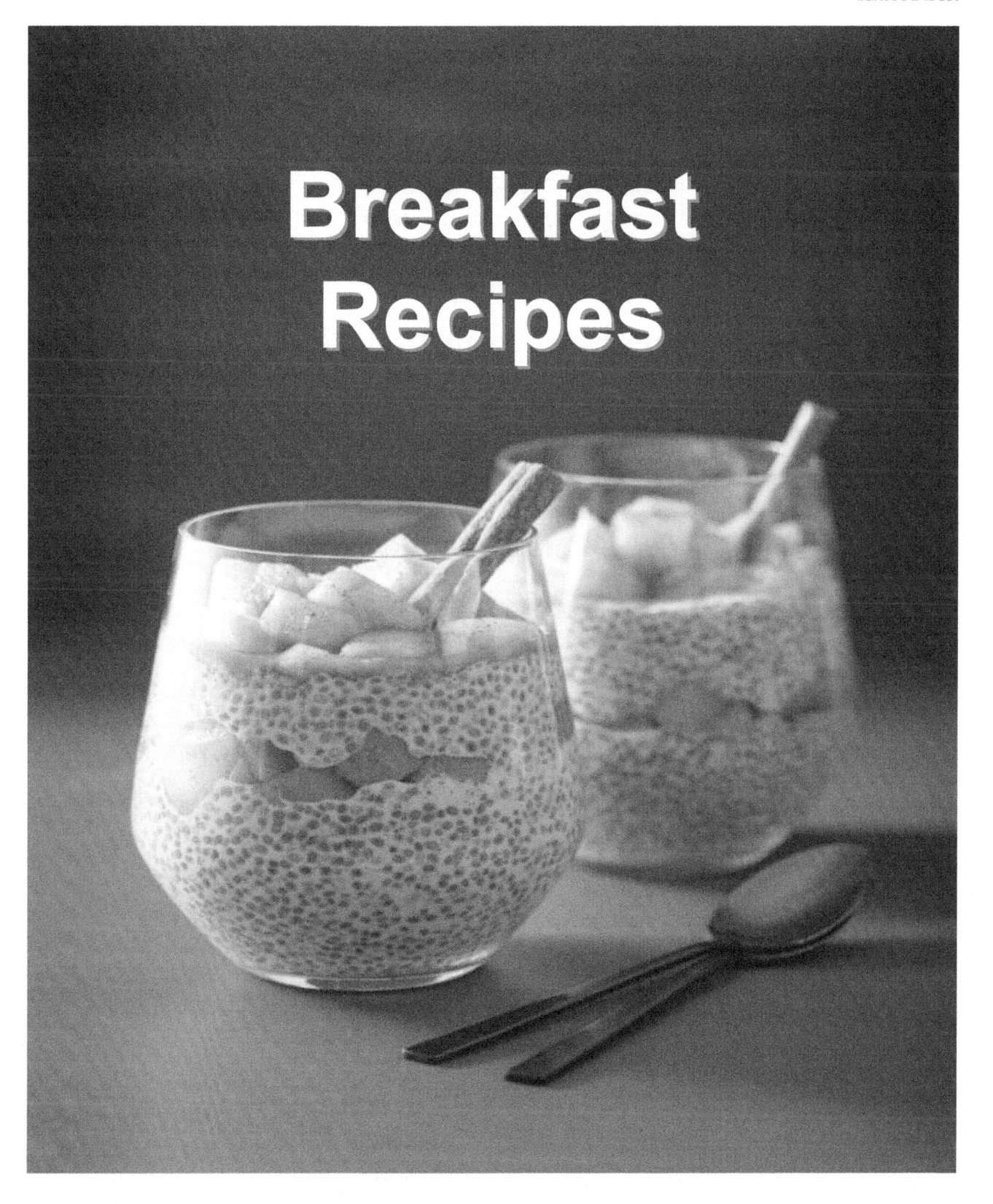

Spinach Porridge

Prep Time 10 Min

Servings 2

Ingredients:
- 2 bunch baby spinach, chopped
- 2 cups walnut milk
- 1 tsp. cinnamon
- 2 tsp. dates syrup

Topping
- Blueberries
- Chia seeds
- Chopped walnuts

Directions:
1. Mix all porridge Ingredients in blender.
2. Pour porridge in bowl.
3. Top with blueberries, baby spinach, chia seeds, and chopped walnuts.
4. Serve and enjoy!

Nutritional information:
Calories Per Servings, 227 kcal, 7.04 g Fat, 36.45 g Total Carbs, 6.95 g Protein, 4.3 g Fiber

Italian Spinach Tofu Omelet

Prep Time 20 min

Servings 2

Ingredients:
- 2 cups baby spinach, finely chopped
- 1 cup, chopped onion
- 1 cup tofu.
- ¼ cup water
- salt & pepper to taste
- 1 tsp. paprika powder
- 1 tsp. oregano
- olive oil for frying

Directions:
1. Blend tofu, salt, pepper, oregano, and paprika in a blender until smooth.
2. Add water slowly in the mixture to make a thick batter.
3. Place a frying pan over medium heat and grease with olive oil.
4. Sautee spinach in pan and cook for 4-5 minutes.
5. Pour tofu mixture in skillet and spread it evenly.
6. Once cooked, flip and cook for another 2-3 minutes.
7. Once the omelet is cooked remove it from heat.
8. Serve hot.
9. Enjoy!

Nutritional information:
Calories Per Servings, 283 kcal, 3.02 g Fat, 57.39 g Total Carbs, 14.52 g Protein, 12.5 g Fiber

Tofu & Arugula Toast

Prep Time 10 min

Servings 4

Ingredients:
- sea salt and black pepper
- 1 tsp. sesame seeds
- 1/4 cup guacamole
- 8 oz. tofu, firm and drained
- 4 slices buckwheat bread
- 1 tbsp. olive oil

Directions:
1. Heat olive oil in pan over medium heat, once the oil is hot, add tofu, fry until golden brown from all sides.
2. Toast bread on a heated griddle for 2-3 minutes per side.
3. Spread guacamole on each bread slice and arrange on a plate.
4. Arrange tofu on bread slice with arugula.
5. Drizzle sesame seeds.
6. Serve and enjoy!

Nutritional information:
Calories Per Servings, 216 kcal, 17.36 g Fat, 8.43 g Total Carbs, 10.45 g Protein, 3.5 g Fiber

Breakfast Tofu Scramble

Prep Time 20 min

Servings 2

Ingredients:
- 1 tablespoon olive oil
- 16 oz. block firm tofu
- 1 teaspoon salt
- 1/4 teaspoon turmeric
- 1/4 teaspoon garlic powder
- 2 tablespoons soy milk

Serving
- 1 buckwheat slice
- Bell pepper.
- Baby spinach leaves

Directions:
1. Heat the olive oil in a pan over medium heat.
2. Crumble the block of tofu right in the pan, with a potato masher or a fork.
3. Cook & stir for 3-4 minutes until the water from the tofu is dried.
4. Add salt, turmeric, and garlic powder.
5. Cook and stir for another 5 minutes.

6. Pour the milk into the pan, and stir to mix. Serve immediately with baby spinach, sauté veggies, and buckwheat leaves.
7. Enjoy!

Nutritional information:
Calories Per Servings, 208 kcal, 15.44 g Fat, 5.45g Total Carbs, 15.2 g Protein, 0.6 g Fiber

Buckwheat& walnuts Pancakes

Prep Time 20 min

Servings 4

Ingredients:
- 1 cup buckwheat flour
- 2 tbsps. dates syrup
- 1 cup soya milk
- 1 tbsps. olive oil
- 2 tablespoons walnut chopped

Directions:
1. Mix all pancake ingredients in a bowl.
2. Heat oil in pan over medium heat. Once the oil is hot pour ¼ cup pancake batter and spread evenly.
3. Cook for 2-3 minutes until golden brown.
4. Flip and cook again.
5. Once cooked remove from heat.
6. Serve with walnuts and dates syrup on top.
7. Enjoy!

Nutritional information:
Calories Per Servings, 197 kcal, 3.92 g Fat, 35.68 g Total Carbs, 7.73 g Protein, 4.43g Fiber

Breakfast Tofu Waffles

Prep Time 10 min

Servings 4

Ingredients:
- 1 cup tofu
- 2 teaspoons baking powder
- 1 teaspoon baking soda
- 1/4 teaspoon salt
- 1/4 teaspoon cinnamon
- 1 1/2 cups soy milk,
- 1 tablespoon apple cider vinegar
- 1/8 cup olive oil

SERVING
- Fresh berries
- Walnut cream
- Chopped walnut

Directions:
1. Mix all waffle ingredients in an electric blender until well incorporated.
2. Preheat a waffle iron and lightly grease with cooking spray.
3. Cook waffles according to the manufacturer's instructions.
4. Serve with fresh berries, walnut cream, and chopped walnut.
5. Enjoy!

Nutritional information:
Calories Per Servings, 260 kcal, 10.27 g Fat, 38.37 g Total Carbs, 7.16 g Protein, 4.7 g Fiber

Savory Buckwheat Porridge

Prep Time 10 min

Servings 4

Ingredients:
- 1 cup buckwheat groats
- 3 cups water
- 1 tablespoon walnut butter
- ½ tablespoon salt
- ½ cup soya milk
- 1 pinch turmeric
- 1 pinch oregano

Directions:
1. In a saucepan bring water to boil.
2. Add buckwheat groats and cook d=covered until cooked through.
3. Turn off heat, add the salt, turmeric, and oregano.
4. Mix well.
5. You can add chopped veggies of your choice.
6. Serve and enjoy!

Nutritional information:
Calories Per Servings, 188 kcal, 4.6 g Fat, 33.56 g Total Carbs, 5.85 g Protein, 4.2 g fiber

French Toast with Berries

Prep Time 10 min

Servings 2

Ingredients:
- 2 slice buckwheat bread
- 2 oz. walnut cream
- 2 tbsps. dates syrup
- Blueberries for serving
- 1 tablespoon walnut butter for toping

Directions:
1. Mix walnut cream and dates syrup in a bowl.
2. Coat bread slice in cream batter and keep it in the freezer for 10 minutes.
3. Grill bread for 2-3 minutes until slices are cooked and brown.
4. Once cooked remove from grill.

5. Serve with fresh blueberries and walnut butter on top.
6. Serve and enjoy!

Nutritional information:
Calories Per Servings, 168 kcal, 7.13 g Fat, 25.45 g Total Carbs, 2.44 g Protein, 2.9 g Fiber

Buckwheat Crepe with Berries

Prep Time 20 min

Servings 4

Ingredients:
- 1 cup buckwheat flour
- 2 tbsps. dates syrup
- 1 cup soy milk
- olive oil
- 1 oz. chocolate syrup
- Fresh berries for topping

Directions:
1. Mix all crepe ingredients in a bowl.
2. Heat oil in pan over medium heat. Once oil is hot pour ¼ cup buckwheat batter and spread evenly.
3. Cook for 2-3 minutes until golden brown.
4. Flip and cook again for 2-3 minutes.
5. Once cooked remove from heat.
6. Serve with fresh berries and chocolate syrup.
7. Serve and enjoy!

Nutritional information:
Calories Per Servings, 121 kcal, 0.49 g Fat, 32.2 g Total Carbs, 0.85 g Protein, 5.3 g Fiber

Kiwi & Apple Porridge

Prep Time 20 min

Servings 2

Ingredients:
- 1 cup buckwheat groats
- 2 cups soy milk
- 2 tablespoons date syrup
- 1 tsp cinnamon
- 1 apple chopped
- 1 kiwi, chopped

Topping
- 1 apple, chopped
- 1 kiwi, sliced
- Fresh blueberries

Directions:
1. Heat pans over medium heat. Add buckwheat and cook for 10 minutes with milk until cooked through.
2. Add cinnamon, chopped apple, and kiwi.
3. Cook for about 8 minutes, then low the heat and then let it leave for 10 minutes.
4. Top with apple slice, kiwi slice, and fresh berries.
5. Enjoy!

Nutritional information:
Calories Per Servings, 292 kcal, 10.15 g Fat, 44 g Total Carbs, 10.7 g Protein, 6.2 g Fiber

Strawberry Smoothie Bowl

Prep Time 5 min

Servings 1

Ingredients:
- 1/2 cup walnut milk
- 1 cup strawberries
- 1 tablespoon dates syrup
- Fresh strawberries for topping
- Chia seeds for topping
- Chopped nuts for topping

Directions:
1. Blend milk, strawberries, and dates syrup in a blender and blend on high speed.
2. Pour the smoothie in a bowl.
3. Top with strawberries, chia seeds, and berries.
4. Serve cool and enjoy!

Nutritional information:
Calories Per Servings, 207 kcal, 10.43 g Fat, 27.1 g Total Carbs, 2.42 g Protein, 1.1 g Fiber

Berries Pancakes

Prep Time 20 min

Servings 4

Ingredients:
- 2 apples, puree
- 1 cup, tofu
- 2 teaspoon baking powder
- 2 tbsps. dates syrup
- ¼ teaspoon salt
- 1 tbsp. olive oil
- 1 cup fresh berries for filling
- ¼ cup dates syrup for topping

Directions:
1. Mix Pancakes Ingredients in blender and mix well.
2. Pour the mixture into a large bowl and fold in half of the berries
3. Heat your skillet over medium heat and grease it with olive oil
4. Pour pancake batter in skillet and spread it slightly.
5. Cook pancake for 2-3 minutes per side, until cooked through.

6. Serve with fresh berries and dates syrup.
7. Enjoy!

Nutritional information:
Calories Per Servings, 211 kcal, 4.62 g Fat, 4.43 g Protein, 42.34 g Total Carbs, 6.5 g Fiber

Walnut Cream Parfait

Prep Time 10 min

Servings 2

Ingredients:
- 1 cup walnut cream
- 1 cup cranberries
- 1 tbsp. dates syrup
- Mint leaves
- 1 tbsp. walnuts, chopped

Directions:
1. Pour walnut cream in serving glass. Add cranberries then pour cream and dates syrup/
2. Top with dates syrup, mint leaves, and walnuts.
3. Serve cold and enjoy!

Nutritional information:
Calories Per Servings, 196 kcal, 2.84 g Fat, 12.48 g Protein, 33.05 g Total Carbs, 1.2 g Fiber

Chocolate Pancakes

Prep Time 20 min

Servings 4

Ingredients:
- 1 cup buckwheat flour
- 2 tbsps. cocoa powder
- 1 tsp baking powder
- 2 tbsp. dates syrup
- 3/4 cup walnut milk
- 1 tsp. olive oil

Directions:
1. Mix all pancake ingredients in a mixing bowl until smooth and well incorporated.
2. Heat nonstick griddle over medium heat, and grease with cooking spray.
3. Pour ¼ batter in griddle and Let it cook for 2-3 minutes until cooked.
4. Flip and cook for another 2-3 minutes until cooked through.
5. Stack the pancakes, drizzle chocolate sauce on top, and fresh strawberries.
6. Enjoy!

Nutritional information:
Calories Per Servings, 169 kcal, 3.57 g Fat, 5.23 g Protein, 31.81 g Total Carbs, 3 g Fiber

Tofu & Spinach Muffins

Prep Time 30 min

Servings 12

Ingredients:
- 1 cup buckwheat flour
- 1 cup tofu, crumbled.
- ¼ cup ground flaxseed
- 2 tsp. baking powder
- ½ tsp salt
- ½ cup walnut milk
- 1 tsp ground cinnamon
- ½ cup dates syrup
- 2 cups spinach, chopped
- ¼ cup walnuts butter

Directions:
1. Preheat oven to 375 degrees F.
2. Mix dry ingredients in a bowl and mix well.
3. Mix wet ingredients in a bowl and mix well.
4. Mix wet ingredients to dry mixture and stir to combine.
5. Carefully add chopped spinach to the batter.
6. Pour batter in lined and greased muffin tins.
7. Bake muffins for about 20-25 until cooked through.
8. Serve hot with green juice and enjoy!

Nutritional information:
Calories Per Servings, 166 kcal, 6.19 g Fat, 3.52 g Protein, 26.94 g Total Carbs, 3.2 g Fiber

Turmeric Tofu Toast

Prep Time 10 min

Servings 4

Ingredients:
- ½ lb. tofu
- 2 onions, sliced
- 1 tsp. garlic, chopped
- 1 tsp turmeric
- 1/8 tsp. pepper & salt
- 2 tbsps. olive oil
- 4 slice buckwheat bread
- chopped parsley for topping

Directions:
1. Heat oil in pan over medium heat, once oil is hot, add garlic and fry.
2. Add onions and fry on low-medium heat for 2-3 minutes.
3. Add crumbled tofu and mash it with a spatula.
4. Season with turmeric, salt, and pepper and mix well.
5. Transfer cooked tofu in plate.
6. Toss bread slice in the same pan.

7. Pour tofu scramble onto warm toast, sprinkle chopped parsley on top.
8. Serve and enjoy!

Nutritional information:
Calories Per Servings, 263 kcal, 18.6 g Fat, 11.78 g Protein, 16.48 g Total Carbs, 4.1 g Fiber

Apple Bread Loaf

Prep Time 60 min

Servings 12

Ingredients:
- 1/4 cup walnut butter, room temperature
- 2 apples, puree
- 2 tbsps. cocoa powder
- 1/4 cup pure dates sugar
- 2 cups buckwheat flour
- 2 tsps. baking powder

Directions:
1. Preheat the oven to 350 degrees F.
2. Grease bread loaf pan with oil and set aside.
3. Mix apple, dates sugar, and butter in a blender and blend.
4. Pour the mixture into a mixing bowl.
5. Add flour, cocoa powder, and baking powder in the bowl and mix well.
6. Pour the batter in greased baking loaf pan.
7. Bake bread for about
8. 40-60 Minutes, or until cooked through.
9. Slice it.
10. Enjoy!

Nutritional information:
Calories Per Servings, 134 kcal, 4.51 g Fat, 2.65 g Protein, 22.71 g Total Carbs, 2.7 g Fiber

Zucchini Tots

Prep Time 40 min

Servings 12

Ingredients:
- 2 cups buckwheat flour
- ¾ cup soy milk
- 1 tsp. baking powder
- ¼ cup walnut butter
- 1 cup broccoli rice
- 1 zucchini, shredded
- ¼ cup chopped walnuts
- 1 tsp. cinnamon powder

Directions:
1. Mix buckwheat flour, walnuts, baking powder, and cinnamon powder in a bowl.
2. Mix milk, butter, zucchini, and broccoli in another bowl,
3. Mix the wet ingredients into the bowl containing the dry ingredients.
4. Preheat the oven to 200 degrees Celsius.
5. Pour batter into each greased muffin cup in the tray.
6. Bake tots for about 20-25 minutes.
7. Once cooked remove from oven.
8. Serve and enjoy!

Nutritional information:
Calories Per Servings, 122 kcal, 5.89 g Fat, 3.22 g Protein, 15.89 g Total Carbs, 2.4 g Fiber

Tofu & Berries Waffles

Prep Time 20 min

Servings 4

Ingredients:
- 1 cup tofu
- ¼ cup walnut butter
- 1/2 cup walnut milk
- ¼ tsp. cinnamon powder
- 2 tbsps. dates syrup
- 1 tsp. baking powder
- Fresh berries for topping

Directions:
1. Turn your waffle maker and set it on medium.
2. Mix all recipe ingredients in blender until smooth and creamy.
3. Pour tofu batter into your waffle maker and cook until the waffle is cooked and crispy.
4. Gently remove the waffles from the machine.
5. Serve with fresh berries on top.
6. Enjoy

Nutritional information:
Calories Per Servings, 231 kcal, 13.46 g Fat, 4.96 g Protein, 25.45 g Total Carbs, 3.4 g Fiber

Chocolate Pudding

Prep Time 30 min

Servings 6

Ingredients:
- 8 slice buckwheat bread
- 1 ½ cups walnut milk
- 2 tbsps. dates syrup
- Dark chocolate for topping

Directions:
1. Blend bread, walnut milk, and dates syrup in blender.
2. Pour the batter into an oven-safe soufflé dish.

3. Cover and steam pudding for 25 minutes on low to medium flame.
4. Once pudding is cooked, remove it from the dish.
5. Pour melted chocolate on top.
6. Freeze for at least 2 hours.
7. Serve and enjoy!

Nutritional information:
Calories Per Servings, 239 kcal, 3.17 g Fat, 8.63 g Protein, 48.19 g Total Carbs, 6.1 g Fiber

Cinnamon & Walnut Tea

Prep Time 5 min

Servings 2

Ingredients:
- 2 cups water
- 1 tsp freshly grated ginger root
- 1/2 tsp ground cinnamon
- 1 tbsp. dates syrup
- ¼ cup walnut milk

Directions:
1. Heat water in a saucepan over medium heat.
2. Add the ginger, ground cinnamon, dates syrup and cook for about 10 minutes.
3. Pour hot walnut milk, once cooked pour in cup
4. Enjoy!

Nutritional information:
Calories Per Servings, 38 kcal, 0.09 g Fat, 0.19 g Protein, 10.16 g Total Carbs, 0.7 g Fiber

Apple Porridge

Prep Time 10 Min

Servings 4

Ingredients:
- 2 apples, chopped
- 3 cups walnut milk
- 1 tsp. cinnamon
- 2 tsp. dates syrup
- TOPPING
- Blueberries
- dark chocolate
- apple slice
- walnuts

Directions:
1. Mix all ingredients in a bowl that fits inside the bowl of your slow cooker.
2. Place the bowl in your slow cooker, and fill your slow cooker with 1 cup of water to surround the bowl.
3. Cook on LOW 6-8 hours, stirring occasionally.
4. Carefully remove the bowl.
5. Top with banana slices and berries.

6. Serve and enjoy!

Nutritional information:
Calories Per Servings, 227 kcal, 7.04 g Fat, 36.45 g Total Carbs, 6.95 g Protein, 4.3 g Fiber

Kale Omelet

Prep Time 20 min

Servings 2

Ingredients:
- 2 cups kale, finely chopped
- 1 cup, chopped onion
- 1 cup buckwheat flour
- ¼ cup water
- salt & pepper to taste
- 1 tsp. paprika powder
- 1 tsp. oregano
- olive oil for frying

Directions:
1. Mix flour, kale, salt, pepper, oregano, and paprika in a bowl and mix well.
2. Add water slowly in the mixture to make a thick batter.
3. Place a frying pan over medium heat and grease with olive oil.
4. Pour ¼ cup mixture in skillet and spread it evenly.
5. Once cooked, flip and cook for another 2-3 minutes.
6. Once the omelet is cooked remove it from heat.
7. Serve with spinach leaves, tomato slices, and cucumber slices.
8. Enjoy!

Nutritional information:
Calories Per Servings, 283 kcal, 3.02 g Fat, 57.39 g Total Carbs, 14.52 g Protein, 12.5 g Fiber

Tofu & Kale Toast

Prep Time 10 min

Servings 4

Ingredients:
- 1 tsp. capers, drained and loosely chopped
- sea salt and black pepper
- 1 tsp. sesame seeds
- 1/4 cup guacamole
- 8 oz. tofu, firm and drained
- 4 slices buckwheat bread
- 4 oz. kale
- 1 tbsp. olive oil

Directions:
1. Heat olive oil in pan over medium heat and fry tofu until golden brown from all sides.
2. Add capers, salt, and pepper to a mixing bowl.
3. Taste and adjust seasonings as needed.

4. Toast bread on a heated griddle for 2-3 minutes per side.
5. Spread guacamole on each bread slice and arrange on a plate.
6. Arrange tofu on bread slice with kale.
7. Drizzle sesame seeds.
8. Serve and enjoy!

Nutritional information:
Calories Per Servings, 216 kcal, 17.36 g Fat, 8.43 g Total Carbs, 10.45 g Protein, 3.5 g Fiber

Tofu Scramble

Prep Time 20 min

Servings 2

Ingredients:
- 1 tablespoon olive oil
- 16 oz. block firm tofu
- 1 teaspoon salt
- 1/4 teaspoon turmeric
- 1/4 teaspoon garlic powder
- 2 tablespoons soy milk

Directions:
1. Heat the olive oil in a pan over medium heat. Mash the block of tofu right in the pan, with a potato masher or a fork.
2. Cook, stirring frequently, for 3-4 minutes until the water from the tofu is dried.
3. Add salt, turmeric, and garlic powder. Cook and stir constantly for about 5 minutes.
4. Pour the milk into the pan, and stir to mix. Serve immediately.
5. Enjoy!

Nutritional information:
Calories Per Servings, 208 kcal, 15.44 g Fat, 5.45g Total Carbs, 15.2 g Protein, 0.6 g Fiber

Buckwheat Pancakes

Prep Time 20 min

Servings 3

Ingredients:
- 1 cup buckwheat flour
- 2 tbsps. dates syrup
- 1 cup soya milk
- 1 tbsps. olive oil

Directions:
1. Mix all ingredients in a bowl.
2. Heat oil in pan over medium heat. Once oil is hot pour ¼ cup buckwheat batter and spread evenly.
3. Cook for 2-3 minutes until golden brown.
4. Flip and cook again.

5. Once cooked remove from heat.
6. Serve and enjoy!

Nutritional information:
Calories Per Servings, 197 kcal, 3.92 g Fat, 35.68 g Total Carbs, 7.73 g Protein, 4.43g Fiber

Waffle Sandwich

Prep Time 10 min

Servings 4

Ingredients:
- 1 1/2 cups buckwheat flour
- 2 teaspoons baking powder
- 1 teaspoon baking soda
- 1/4 teaspoon salt
- 1/4 teaspoon cinnamon, optional
- 1 1/2 cups soy milk,
- 1 tablespoon apple cider vinegar
- 1/8 cup olive oil
  SERVING
- lettuce leaves
- cucumber slice

Directions:
1. Mix all ingredients in a bowl until well incorporated.
2. Preheat a waffle iron and lightly grease with cooking spray. Cook waffles according to the manufacturer's instructions.
3. Serve with lettuce leaves and cucumber slice between two waffles.
4. Enjoy!

Nutritional information:
Calories Per Servings, 260 kcal, 10.27 g Fat, 38.37 g Total Carbs, 7.16 g Protein, 4.7 g Fiber

Buckwheat Porridge

Prep Time 10 min

Servings 4

Ingredients:
- 1 cup buckwheat groats
- 1 cup chopped kale
- 3 cups water
- 1 tablespoon walnut butter
- ½ tablespoon salt
- ½ cup soya milk
- 1 teaspoon dates syrup

Directions:
1. In a saucepan bring water to boil.
2. Add uncooked buckwheat groats. Cover the pot and simmer for 10 minutes (or until water is absorbed).

3. Turn off heat, add the salt, chopped kale, dates syrup and let it sit for 10 more minutes.
4. Top with butter and serve warm in a savory dish, or as a porridge with milk and toppings.

Nutritional information:
Calories Per Servings, 188 kcal, 4.6 g Fat, 33.56 g Total Carbs, 5.85 g Protein, 4.2 g Fiber

Toast with Caramelized Apple

Prep Time 10 min

Servings 2

Ingredients:
- 2 slice buckwheat bread slices 2 oz. chocolate cream
- 1 cup apple
- 2 tbsps. dates syrup
- 1/2 cup water

Directions:
1. Grill bread for 2 minutes.
2. Heat water in a pan over medium heat.
3. Add dates syrup and apple and cook for 5-8 minutes until apples are soft and caramelize.
4. Spread chocolate cream over the grill bread slice.
5. Sprinkle caramelize apple on top.
6. Serve and enjoy!

Nutritional information:
Calories Per Servings, 168 kcal, 7.13 g Fat, 25.45 g Total Carbs, 2.44 g Protein, 2.9 g Fiber

Buckwheat Crepe with Apple

Prep Time 20 min

Servings 4

Ingredients:
- 1 cup buckwheat flour
- 2 tbsps. dates syrup
- 1 cup soy milk
- olive oil
- 2 oz. Caramelized apple

Directions:
1. Mix all ingredients in a bowl.
2. Heat oil in pan over medium heat. Once oil is hot pour ¼ cup buckwheat batter and spread evenly.
3. Cook for 2-3 minutes until golden brown.
4. Flip and cook again.
5. Once cooked remove from heat.
6. Wrap with caramelized apple.
7. Serve and enjoy!

Nutritional information:
Calories Per Servings, 121 kcal, 0.49 g Fat, 32.2 g Total Carbs, 0.85 g Protein, 5.3 g Fiber

Buckwheat & Apple Porridge

Prep Time 20 min

Servings 2

Ingredients:
- 1 cup buckwheat groats
- 2 cups soy milk
- pinch of salt
- 1 tsp cinnamon
- 1 sour apple
- Topping
- 1 apple, chopped
- 1 oz. walnuts

Directions:
1. Bring milk to a boil, season lightly with salt, and add buckwheat groats.
2. Add cinnamon to taste, and a grated sour apple.
3. Cook for about 8 minutes, then low the heat and let the buckwheat rest in a covered pot for another 10 minutes.
4. Serve the buckwheat porridge with apple and walnut topping.
5. Enjoy!

Nutritional information:
Calories Per Servings, 292 kcal, 10.15 g Fat, 44 g Total Carbs, 10.7 g Protein, 6.2 g Fiber

Acai Berry Smoothie Bowl

Prep Time 5 min

Servings 1

Ingredients:
- 1/2 cup walnut milk
- 1 cup acai berry
- 1/4 tsp salt
- Fresh berries for topping

Directions:
1. Blend milk, berries salt, in a blender, and blend on high speed.
2. Pour the smoothie in a bowl.
3. Top with raspberries, blueberries.
4. Serve cool and enjoy!

Nutritional information:
Calories Per Servings, 207 kcal, 10.43 g Fat, 27.1 g Total Carbs, 2.42 g Protein, 1.1 g Fiber

Walnuts Porridge

Prep Time 20 Min

Servings 2

Ingredients:
- 1 cup soy milk
- 1 date, chopped
- 2 tbsps. buckwheat flakes
- 1 tsp. walnut butter
- 1 green apple slices
- 2 oz. pomegranate seeds
- 1 /2 oz. walnuts

Directions:
1. Place the milk and dates in a pan over medium heat.
2. Add the buckwheat flakes, walnuts and cook for 10 minutes.
3. Once porridge is cooked remove from heat.
4. Serve with apple slice, pomegranate seeds, and walnuts on top.
5. Enjoy!

Nutritional information:
Ca Calories Per Servings, 278 kcal, 11.39 g Fat, 7.28 g Protein, 41.29 g Total Carbs, 5.7 g Fiber

Apple Pancakes

Prep Time 20 min

Servings 4

Ingredients:
- 2 apples, puree
- 1 cup, buckwheat flour
- 2 tsp baking powder
- 2 tbsps. dates syrup
- ¼ teaspoon salt
- 1 tbsp. olive oil
- 1 cup blueberries
- 2-3 strawberries, sliced

Directions:
1. Mix apple puree, flour, baking powder, dates syrup, and salt to the blender and blend for 2 minutes.
2. Pour the mixture into a large bowl and fold in half of the blueberries.
3. Heat your skillet over medium heat and grease it with olive oil
4. Pour ¼ cup pancake batter in skillet and spread it slightly.
5. Cook pancake for 2-3 minutes per side, until cooked through.
6. Serve with berries.
7. Enjoy!

Nutritional information:

Calories Per Servings, 211 kcal, 4.62 g Fat, 4.43 g Protein, 42.34 g Total Carbs, 6.5 g Fiber

Morning Parfait

Prep Time 10 min

Servings 2

Ingredients:
- 1 cup soy yogurt
- 1 cup cranberries
- 1 tbsp. dates syrup
- Mint leaves
- 1 tbsp. walnuts, chopped

Directions:
1. Pour 2 tbsps. soy yogurt in serving glass. then layer with cranberries.
2. Repeat with layer.
3. Top with dates syrup, mint leaves, and walnuts.
4. Serve cold and enjoy!

Nutritional information:
Calories Per Servings, 196 kcal, 2.84 g Fat, 12.48 g Protein, 33.05 g Total Carbs, 1.2 g Fiber

Spinach Muffins

Prep Time 30 min

Servings 12

Ingredients:
- 2 cups buckwheat flour
- ¼ cup ground flaxseed
- 2 tsp. baking powder
- ½ tsp salt½ cup soy milk
- 1 tsp ground cinnamon
- ½ cup dates syrup
- 2 cups spinach, chopped
- ¼ cup walnuts butter

Directions:
1. Preheat oven to 375 degrees F.
2. Mix dry ingredients in a bowl and mix well.
3. Mix wet ingredients in a bowl and mix well.
4. Mix wet ingredients to dry mixture and stir to combine.
5. Carefully mix chopped spinach in batter.
6. Pour batter in lined and greased muffin tins.
7. Bake muffins for about 20-25 minutes or until toothpick comes out clean.
8. Serve hot with green tea and enjoy!

Nutritional information:
Calories Per Servings, 166 kcal, 6.19 g Fat, 3.52 g Protein, 26.94 g Total Carbs, 3.2 g Fiber

Chocolate Pancakes

Prep Time 20 min

Servings 4

Ingredients:
- 1 cup buckwheat flour
- 2 tbsps. cocoa powder
- 1 tsp baking powder
- 2 tbsp. dates syrup
- 3/4 cup soy milk
- 1 tsp. olive oil

Directions:
1. Mix buckwheat flour, baking powder, and cocoa powder in a mixing bowl.
2. Add dates syrup, milk, and oil and mix well.
3. Heat nonstick griddle over medium heat, and grease with cooking spray.
4. Pour ¼ batter in griddle and Let it cook for 2-3 minutes until cooked.
5. Flip and cook for another 2-3 minutes until cooked through.
6. Stack the pancakes, drizzle chocolate syrup on top, and banana slice.
7. Enjoy!

Buckwheat Bread Loaf

Prep Time 60 min

Servings 12

Ingredients:
- 1/4 cup melted walnut butter
- 2 apples, puree
- 1/4 cup pure dates syrup
- 2 cups buckwheat flour
- 2 tsps. baking powder

Directions:
1. Preheat the oven to 350 degrees F.
2. Grease an 8-inch loaf pan with coconut oil and set aside.
3. Mix apple, dates syrup, and butter in a blender and blend.
4. Pour the mixture into a mixing bowl.
5. Add flour and baking powder in a bowl and mix well.
6. Pour the batter in greased baking loaf pan.
7. Bake for 40-60 Minutes, or until cooked through.
8. Allow to cool before cutting.
9. Enjoy!

Nutritional information:
Calories Per Servings, 134 kcal, 4.51 g Fat, 2.65 g Protein, 22.71 g Total Carbs, 2.7 g Fiber

Broccoli Muffins

Prep Time 40 min

Servings 12

Ingredients:
- 2 cups buckwheat flour
- ¾ cup soy milk
- ¼ cup walnut butter
- 1 cup broccoli, roughly chopped
- 4-8 strawberries, sliced
- ¼ cup chopped walnuts
- 1 tsp. cinnamon powder

Directions:
1. Mix buckwheat flour, walnuts, and cinnamon powder in a bowl.
2. Mix milk, butter, strawberries, and broccoli in another bowl,
3. Gently pour the wet ingredients into the bowl containing the dry ingredients.
4. Preheat the oven to 200 degrees Celsius.
5. Line muffin tray with paper liners.
6. Pour batter into each muffin cup in the tray.
7. Bake for about 20-25 minutes.
8. Once cooked remove from oven.
9. Serve and enjoy!

Nutritional information:
Calories Per Servings, 122 kcal, 5.89 g Fat, 3.22 g Protein, 15.89 g Total Carbs, 2.4 g Fiber

Buckwheat Waffles

Prep Time 20 min

Servings 4

Ingredients:
- 1 cup buckwheat flour
- ¼ cup walnut butter
- 1/2 cup soy milk
- ¼ tsp. cinnamon powder
- 2 tbsps. dates syrup
- 1 tsp. baking powder

Directions:
1. Turn your waffle maker and set it on medium.
2. Mix all recipe ingredients in a bowl and mix well.
3. Pour this batter into your waffle maker and cook until the waffle is cooked and crispy.
4. Gently remove the waffles from the machine.
5. Serve with walnut butter on top.
6. Enjoy!

Nutritional information:
Calories Per Servings, 231 kcal, 13.46 g Fat, 4.96 g Protein, 25.45 g Total Carbs, 3.4 g Fiber

Eggless Pudding

Prep Time 30 min

Servings 6

Ingredients:
- 8 slice buckwheat bread
- 1 ½ cups soy milk
- 2 tbsps. dates syrup
- 3 tbsps. dates sugar
- 1 tbsps. walnut butter

Directions:
1. Blend bread, milk, and dates syrup in blender.
2. Add sugar with butter in a pan and place it on medium to high heat.
3. Allow sugar to melt and turn golden.
4. Transfer the caramel into an oven-safe soufflé dish and fill the dish with the bread mixture.
5. Cover with an aluminum wrap and steam for 25 minutes on low to medium flame.
6. Once cooked remove from dish.
7. Refrigerate for at least 2 hours.
8. Serve and enjoy!

Nutritional information:
Calories Per Servings, 239 kcal, 3.17 g Fat, 8.63 g Protein, 48.19 g Total Carbs, 6.1 g Fiber

Turmeric Tea

Prep Time 5 min

Servings 2

Ingredients:
- 2 cups water
- 1 tsp freshly grated turmeric root
- 1 tsp freshly grated ginger root
- 1/2 tsp ground cinnamon
- 1 tbsp. dates syrup

Directions:
1. Place water in a saucepan and heat over medium.
2. Add the turmeric root, ginger, ground cinnamon, and dates syrup, and cook for 10 minutes.
3. Once cooked pour in glass.
4. Enjoy!

Nutritional information:
Calories Per Servings, 38 kcal, 0.09 g Fat, 0.19 g Protein, 10.16 g Total Carbs, 0.7 g Fiber

Buckwheat Granola

Prep Time 5 min

Servings 2

Ingredients:
- 2 cups raw buckwheat groats
- ¾ cup pumpkin seeds
- ¾ cup almonds, chopped
- 1 cup unsweetened coconut flakes
- 1 teaspoon ground cinnamon
- 1 teaspoon ground ginger
- 1 ripe banana, peeled
- 2 tablespoons maple syrup
- 2 tablespoons extra-virgin olive oil

Directions:
1. Preheat the oven to 350 degrees F.
2. In a bowl, place the buckwheat groats, coconut flakes pumpkin seeds, almonds, and spices and mix well.
3. In another bowl, add the banana, and with a fork, mash well.
4. Add to the buckwheat mixture, maple syrup, and oil and mix until well combined.
5. Transfer the mixture onto the prepared baking sheet and spread in an even layer.
6. Bake for about 25-30 minutes, stirring once halfway through.
7. Remove the baking sheet from the oven and set aside to cool.

Nutritional information:
Calories Per Servings, 252 kcal, 14g Fat, 7 g Protein, 26 g Total Carbs, 4 g Fiber

Chocolate Granola

Prep Time 30 min

Servings 8

Ingredients:
- ¼ cup cacao powder
- ¼ cup maple syrup
- 2 tablespoons coconut oil, melted
- ½ teaspoon vanilla extract
- 1/8 teaspoon salt
- 2 cups gluten-free rolled oats
- ¼ cup unsweetened coconut flakes
- 2 tablespoons chia seeds
- 2 tablespoons unsweetened dark chocolate, chopped finely

Directions:
1. Preheat the oven to 300 degrees F. Line a medium baking sheet with parchment paper.
2. In a medium pan, add the cacao powder, maple syrup, coconut oil, vanilla extract, and salt and mix well.
3. Now, place pan over medium heat and cook for about 2-3 minutes or until thick and syrupy, stirring continuously.
4. Remove from the heat and set aside.
5. In a large bowl, add the oats, coconut, and chia seeds and mix well.

6. Add the syrup mixture and mix until well combined.
7. Transfer the granola mixture onto a prepared baking sheet and spread in an even layer.
8. Bake for about 35 minutes.
9. Remove from the oven and set aside for about 1 hour.
10. Add the chocolate pieces and stir to combine.
11. Serve immediately.

Nutritional information:
Calories Per Servings, 193 kcal, 9 g Fat, 5 g Protein, 26 g Total Carbs, 4 g Fiber

Buckwheat Porridge with berries

Prep Time 30 min

Servings 2

Ingredients:
- 1 cup buckwheat, rinsed
- 1 cup unsweetened almond milk
- 1 cup water
- ½ teaspoon ground cinnamon
- ½ teaspoon vanilla extract
- 1-2 tablespoons raw honey
- ¼ cup fresh blueberries

Directions:
1. In a pan, add all the ingredients except honey and blueberries over medium-high heat and bring to a boil.
2. Reduce the heat to low and simmer, covered for about 10 minutes.
3. Stir in the honey and remove from the heat.
4. Set aside, covered, for about 5 minutes with a fork, fluff the mixture and transfer into serving bowls.
5. Top with blueberries and serve.

Nutritional information:
Calories Per Servings, 38 kcal, 0.09 g Fat, 0.19 g Protein, 10.16 g Total Carbs, 0.7 g Fiber

Blueberry Pancakes

Prep Time 30 min

Servings 8

Ingredients:
- ½ cup walnut milk
- 1 tablespoon coconut oil
- 1 egg, beaten lightly
- 1/3 cup buckwheat flour
- 1 teaspoon baking powder
- Pinch of salt
- ¼ cup frozen blueberries

Directions:

1. Put all ingredients except berries in a mixing bowl and mix thoroughly.
2. Fold in blueberries.
3. Heat a greased non-stick skillet over medium heat.
4. Place 2 tbsps. of the mixture and spread in an even circle.
5. Cook for about 2-3 minutes.
6. Flip and cook for an additional 1 minute.
7. Repeat with the remaining mixture.
8. Serve warm.

Nutritional information:
Calories Per Servings, 38 kcal, 0.09 g Fat, 0.19 g Protein, 10.16 g Total Carbs, 0.7 g Fiber

Pumpkin Pancakes

Prep Time 30 min

Servings 8

Ingredients:
- 2 tablespoons ground flaxseed
- 6 tablespoons filtered water
- 1 cup buckwheat flour
- 1 tablespoon baking powder
- 1 teaspoon pumpkin pie spice
- ½ teaspoon salt
- 1 cup pumpkin puree
- ¾ cup plus 2 tablespoons unsweetened almond milk
- 3 tablespoons pure maple syrup
- 2 tablespoons coconut oil
- 1 teaspoon vanilla extract

Directions:
1. In a bowl, add ground flaxseed and mix well. Set aside for about 5 minutes or until thickened.
2. In a blender, add flaxseed mixture and remaining ingredients and pulse until well combined.
3. Transfer the mixture into a bowl and set aside for about 10 minutes.
4. Heat a greased non-stick skillet over medium heat.
5. Place about ¼ cup of the mixture and spread in an even circle.
6. Cook for about 2 minutes per side.
7. Repeat with the remaining mixture.
8. Serve warm.

Nutritional information:
Calories Per Servings, 102 kcal, 4 g Fat, 0.19 g Protein, 15 g Total Carbs, 2 g Fiber

Matcha Pancakes

Prep Time 30 min
Servings 8

Ingredients:
- 2 tablespoons flax meal
- 5 tablespoons warm water
- 1 cup spelt flour
- 1 cup buckwheat flour
- 1 tablespoon matcha powder
- 1 tablespoon baking powder
- Pinch of salt
- ¾ cup unsweetened almond milk
- 1 tablespoon extra-virgin olive oil
- 1 teaspoon vanilla extract
- 1/3 cup raw honey

Directions:
1. In a bowl, add the flax meal and warm water and mix well. Set aside for about 5 minutes.
2. In another bowl, place the flours, matcha powder, baking powder, and salt and mix well.
3. In the bowl of flax meal mixture, place the almond milk, oil, and vanilla extract and beat until well combined.
4. Now, place the flour mixture and mix until a smooth textured mixture is formed.
5. Heat a lightly greased non-stick wok over medium-high heat.
6. Add desired amount of mixture and with a spoon, spread into an even layer.
7. Cook for about 2-3 minutes.
8. Carefully, flip the side and cook for aBOUT1 minute.
9. Repeat with the remaining mixture.

Nutritional information:
Calories Per Servings, 232 kcal, 0.6 g Fat, 0.19 g Protein, 10.16 g Total Carbs, 0.7 g Fiber

Overnight Oat Pudding

Prep Time 5 min
Cooking time 10 min
Total time 15 min
Servings 4

Ingredients:
- 1 banana
- 3/4 cup walnut milk
- 2 tbsps. dates syrup
- Pinch sea salt
- 1 cup rolled oats
- 1 1/2 tbsps. chia seeds
- 1 cup strawberries sliced

Directions:
1. Blend the banana, almond milk, dates, and sea salt in a blender till smooth.
2. Place the oats and chia seeds in an airtight container. Pour the liquid mixture over the oats and chia seeds and mix well.
3. Cover and refrigerate overnight.
4. In the morning, mix again and add some milk.
5. Top with fresh strawberries slice and enjoy.

Zucchini And Chickpeas Frittata

Prep Time 10 min
Cooking time 30 min
Total time 40 min
Servings 8

INGREDIENTS
- 1 cup coconut milk
- 1 cup chickpeas flour
- 1 tsp. dried oregano
- Salt and pepper, to taste
- 4-6 baby zucchini
- 1 tsp. baking powder
- 4-5 zucchini flowers
- ½ cup thinly sliced red onion
- 1 tsp. olive oil

Directions:
1. Heat oil in a pan over medium heat.
2. Once the oil is hot, add onion and cook for 2-3 minutes.
3. Add zucchini and cook for 4-5 minutes.
4. Add zucchini and onion in greased casserole pan.
5. Mix chickpeas with milk in a bowl with baking powder, salt, pepper, and oregano.
6. Pour this batter over zucchini, top with zucchini flowers.
7. Bake in preheated oven for about 20-30 minutes until cooked through.
8. Serve hot and enjoy!

Walnuts Pudding With Oats

Prep Time 5 min
Cooking time min
Total time 5 min
Servings 4

Ingredients:
- 1/2 cup oats rolled oats
- 1/4 cup chia seeds
- 1 cup walnut milk
- pinch of salt
- 1 tbsp. dates syrup
- 1 cup strawberries

- yogurt for topping
- berries for topping
- walnuts for topping

Directions:
1. Place the oats, seeds, milk, salt, dates syrup in a jar with a lid. Refrigerate overnight.
2. In the morning set strawberries on the wall of the serving jar.
3. Pour oats mixture.
4. Top with oats, strawberries, and chopped walnuts.
5. Serve and enjoy!

Homemade walnut Bagels

Prep Time 10 min
Cooking time 30 min
Total time 40 min
Servings 4

Ingredients:
- 1 cup plain, walnut cream
- 1 cup buckwheat flour
- 2 tsp. baking powder
- ¼ tsp salt
- 1 tsp. sesame seeds

Directions:
1. Preheat oven to 400°F.
2. Mix flour, salt, and baking powder in a bowl.
3. Add yogurt and make the thick dough and knead the dough for about 30 seconds.
4. Cut the dough into 4 equal parts and roll each dough piece into a ball and create a hole in the center and stretch it.
5. Place bagels on a prepared baking sheet.
6. Brush egg over the bagels and drizzle sesame seeds on top.
7. Bake for about 25-30 minutes.
8. Once cooked remove from heat.
9. Cut bagels in half and spread coconut cream.

Kale & Buckwheat Pancakes

Prep Time 10 min
Cooking time 20 min
Total time 30 min
Servings 4

Ingredients:
- 1 cup, chopped onion
- 1 cup chopped kale
- 1 cup buckwheat, flour
- ¼ cup water
- salt & pepper to taste
- 1 tsp. mustard powder
- 1 tsp. paprika powder
- olive oil for frying
- walnut cream for topping

Directions:
1. Mix all ingredients in a bowl and add water slowly to make a thick batter.
2. Heat oil in a pan over medium heat.
3. Once the oil is hot pour 2-3 tbsps. of batter and slightly spread it.
4. Cook for 2-3 minutes over medium heat.
5. Once cooked, flip and cook for another 2-3 minutes.
6. Serve with arugula leaves, tomato slice, and coconut cream.
7. Enjoy!

Frutti & Nutty Breakfast Bowl

Prep Time 10 min
Cooking time 00 min
Total time 10 min
Servings 2

Ingredients:
- 4 oz. walnuts
- 1 kiwi fruit, sliced
- 1 orange, sliced
- 1 cup fresh berries
- 1 cup walnut cream

Directions:
1. Pour walnuts, berries, kiwi, orange slices, and walnut cream in a serving bowl.
2. Top with mint leaves.
3. Enjoy!

Pumpkin Porridge

Prep Time 10 min
Cooking time 20 min
Total time 30 min
Servings 4

Ingredients:
- 1 lb. pumpkin, chopped
- 4 cups water
- 1 pinch salt
- 1 tbsp. olive oil

Directions:
1. Pour water, pumpkin, salt, and oil in a pan and cook over medium heat.
2. Cook porridge for about 25-30.
3. Once cooked and water is dried remove from heat.
4. Serve and enjoy!

Creamy Oat Porridge

Prep Time 10 min
Cooking time 20 min
Total time 30 min

Servings 2

Ingredients:
- 1 cup walnut milk
- 1/2 cup roll oats
- 2 tbsps. maple syrup

Topping
- 1 kiwi sliced
- 2 oz. walnuts
- 1 tsp. flax seeds
- 1 oz. pumpkin seeds
- mint leaves

Directions:
1. Heat your saucepan over medium heat.
2. Pour oats, milk, and maple syrup, cook over medium heat for about 10-15 minutes until cooked through.
3. Pour cooked porridge in a serving bowl and let it cool at room temperature.
4. Top it with a kiwi slice, walnuts, flax seeds, pumpkin seeds, and mint leaves.
5. Enjoy!

Kale Muffins

Prep Time: 10 min
Cooking Time: 25 min
Total Time: 35 min

Servings: 6

Ingredients:
- 1 cup chopped kale
- 1 cup buckwheat flour
- 1 tbsp. maple syrup
- ¼ cup walnut milk
- 1 tsp. baking powder
- ¼ cup chopped dates
- ¼ cup olive oil
- ¼ tsp. ground cinnamon

Directions:
1. Mix flour, baking powder, syrup, milk oil, and cinnamon powder in a bowl.
2. Fold in the dates and kale.
3. Preheat the oven.
4. Grease a muffin tray and add 2 tbsps. of the batter in each greased cup.
5. Bake muffins for about 25 minutes at 350 degrees Celsius.
6. once cooked remove from oven.
7. Serve and enjoy!

Dates & Oats Bars

Prep Time 15 Min
Cooking Time 20 Min
Total Time 35 Min

Servings: 16

Ingredients:
- 1 1/2 cup oats
- 1/2 cup buckwheat flour
- 16 oz. Medjool dates
- 1/2 cup walnuts
- ¼ cup maple syrup
- 2 tbsps. ground flax
- 1/4 cup coconut oil
- 1 tsp. lemon juice

Directions:
1. Preheat oven to 325º F.
2. Mix oats, buckwheat flour, dates, walnuts, ground flax, coconut oil, maple syrup, and lemon juice in the processor bowl, and process until all ingredients are mixed.
3. Line an 8 x 8 pan with baking paper.
4. Pour the mixture into a pan and level it with a spatula.
5. Bake pan in preheated oven for about 20 minutes.
6. Once cooked remove from oven.
7. Let it stand at room temperature.

Chocolate Tea Latte

Prep Time 10 Min
Cooking Time 10 Min
Total Time 20 Min

Servings 4

Ingredients:
- 2 cinnamon sticks, broken into pieces
- 2 tsps. whole black peppercorns
- 10 whole cloves
- 6 green cardamom pods, cracked
- 4 cups water
- 1-piece fresh ginger, thinly sliced
- 2 tbsps. loose-leaf black tea
- ½ cup maple syrup
- 2 cups walnut milk
- 2 tbsp. cocoa powder

Directions:
1. Toss cinnamon, peppercorns, cloves, cocoa powder, and cardamom in a small saucepan over medium for about 3 to 4 minutes.
2. Add water and ginger and bring to a simmer for about 5 minutes.

3. Remove from the heat and add loose-leaf tea. Cover and steep for 10 minutes.
4. Add maple syrup and mix well.
5. Add milk and cook again on low heat for 5-8 minutes.
6. Strain the tea.
7. Pour in cup, sprinkle cinnamon powder on top.
8. Enjoy!

No Bake Brownies Bites

Prep Time: 10 min
Cooking Time: 10 min
Total Time: 20 min

Servings: 6

Ingredients:
- 1/2 cup walnuts, chopped
- 1/2 cup buckwheat flour
- 1 cup dates, chopped
- 1/3 cup cocoa powder
- 1/2 cup coconut flour
- ¼ cup sesame seeds

Directions:
1. Grind the walnuts, buckwheat, and coconut in a food processor, until mix together.
2. Add the dates, cocoa powder, and mix again.
3. Roll the mixture into round balls. Roll the balls on the sesame seeds.
4. Place brownies bite in the fridge for about 2 hours until set.
5. Serve and enjoy!

Kiwi Fruit Pudding

Prep Time 10 min
Cooking time 00 min
Total time 10 min

Servings 2

Ingredients:
- 1 cup kiwi fruit puree
- 1 cup walnut cream
- 1 cup fresh strawberries

Directions:
1. Pour ¼ cup cream into 2 serving glasses.
2. Pour kiwi puree over cream and layer of strawberries on each serving glass.
3. Serve and enjoy!

Baked French Toast with Berries

Prep Time 15 Min
Cooking time 25 Min
Total time 40 Min

Servings 8

Ingredients:
- 8 buckwheat bread slices
- 1 small ripe banana
- 1/2 cup walnut milk
- 2 tbsps. maple syrup
- 2 tbsps. buckwheat flour
- 1 tsp. olive oil
- pinch of cinnamon
- berries for topping

Directions:
1. Blend ripe banana, milk, flour, maple syrup, buckwheat flour, oil, and cinnamon powder in blender and transfer to a shallow bowl.
2. Bake in the oven for about 10-20 minutes until crispy.
3. Once cooked arrange in a plate, top with berries and enjoy!

Kale & Chickpeas Omelet

Prep Time 10 min
Cooking time 20 min
Total time 30 min

Servings 4

Ingredients:
- 2 cups kale, finely chopped
- 1 cup, chopped onion
- 1 cup chickpeas, flour
- ¼ cup water
- salt & pepper to taste
- 1 tsp. paprika powder
- olive oil for frying

Directions:
1. Mix chickpeas flour, kale, salt, pepper, and paprika in a bowl and mix well.
2. Add water slowly in the mixture to make a thick batter.
3. Place a frying pan over medium heat and grease with olive oil.
4. Pour ¼ cup mixture in skillet and spread it evenly.
5. Once cooked, flip and cook for another 2-3 minutes.
6. Once the omelet is cooked remove it from heat.
7. Serve with spinach leaves, tomato slices, and cucumber slices.
8. Enjoy!

Savory Zucchini Pancakes

Prep Time 10 min
Cooking time 20 min
Total time 30 min

Servings 6

Ingredients:

- 2 cups zucchini, grated and squeezed
- 1 onion, chopped
- 1 cup buckwheat, flour
- ¼ cup water
- salt & pepper to taste
- 1 tsp. paprika powder
- olive oil for frying

Directions:
1. Mix zucchini, onion, buckwheat flour, salt, pepper, and paprika in a bowl and mix well.
2. Add water slowly in a mixture to make a thick batter.
3. Place skillet over medium heat and grease with olive oil.

Kale & Buckwheat Breakfast Bowl

Prep Time 5 min
Cooking time 15 min
Total time 20 min

Servings 4

Ingredients:
- 1 tsp. onion powder
- ½ tsp. salt
- ½ tsp. pepper
- 1 tsp. olive oil
- 1 bag baby kale
- 1 cup buckwheat, groats
- 1 cup cooked quinoa
- 1 carrot, sliced and steamed
- 1 tsp. sesame seeds

Directions:

1. Mix carrots, quinoa, and groats in a bowl.
2. Mix onion powder, salt, pepper, and oil in a bowl and mix with chickpeas mix.
3. Drizzle sesame seeds on top.
4. Serve with kale and enjoy it!
5. Pour ¼ cup mixture in skillet and cook over medium heat for 2-3 minutes.
6. Once cooked, flip and cook for another 2-3 minutes.
7. Once cooked remove from heat.
8. Serve hot and enjoy!

Muesli Breakfast Bowl with Berries

Prep Time 10 min
Cooking time 20 min
Total time 30 min

Servings: 2

Ingredients:
- 1 cup muesli
- 2/3 cup coconut milk
- 1/4 cup blueberries
- 1 apple sliced with skin
- 1 oz. roasted pumpkin seeds

Directions:
1. Add 1 cup muesli to a medium-sized bowl with milk and soak for about 20 minutes or overnight.
2. Once tender and soft.
3. Serve soaked muesli with an apple slice, blueberries, pumpkin seeds.

Serve and enjoy!

Green Salads Recipes

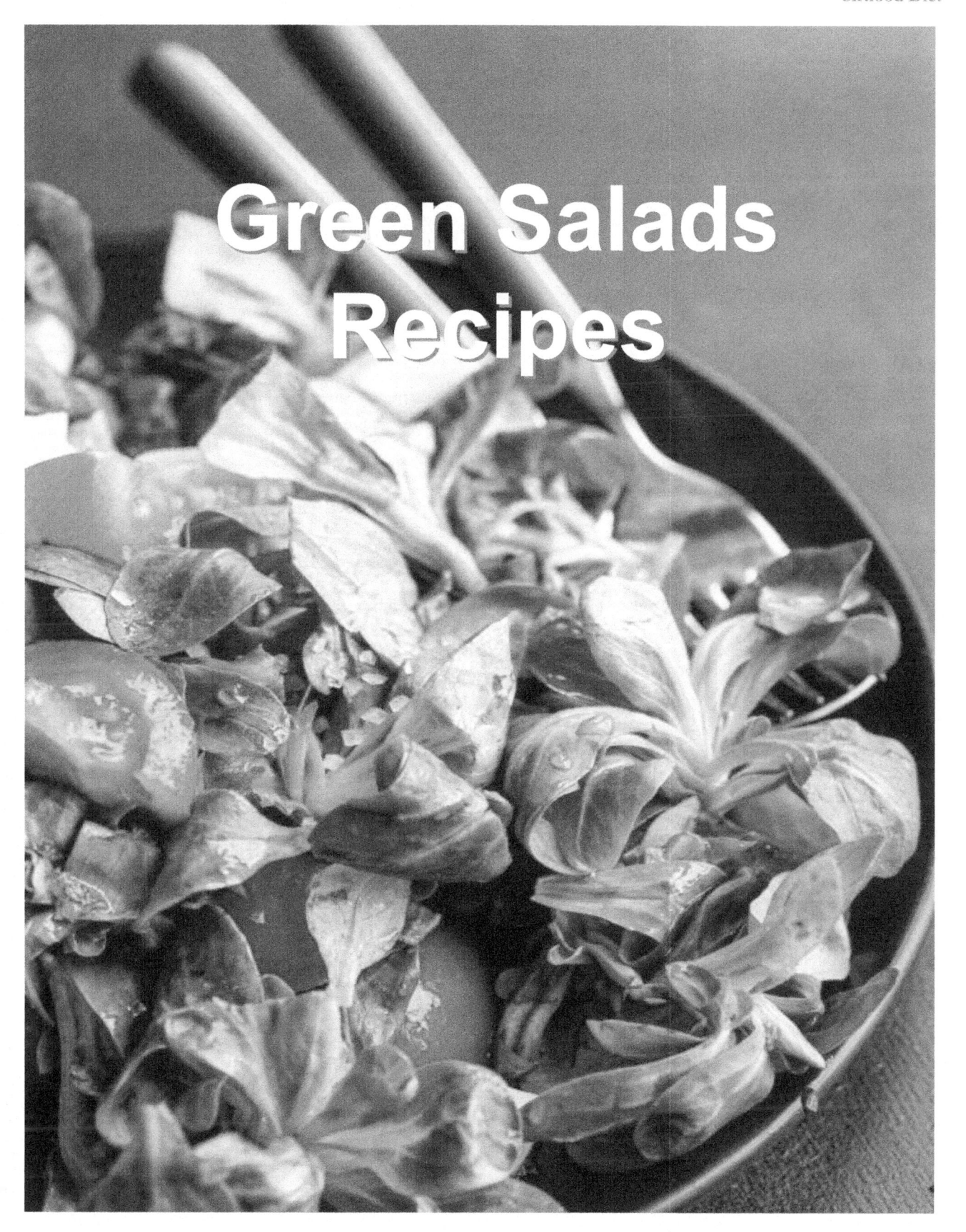

Green Veggies Salad Bowl

Prep Time 10 min

Servings 2

Ingredients:
- 1 red onion, sliced
- 1 bunch parsley leaves
- 1 bunch arugula leaves.
- 1 cucumber, chopped
- 1 bunch spinach, chopped
- 2-3 tomatoes, sliced

DRESSING
- ¼ cup lemon juice
- 1 tbsp. olive oil
- Salt & pepper to taste
- 1 tsp garlic powder.

Directions:
1. Mix all dressing ingredients in a bowl and set aside.
2. Cut and chop veggies and pour them into the bowl.
3. Drizzle and mix dressing over veggies.
4. Slightly mix.
5. Serve and enjoy!

Nutritional information:
Calories Per Servings, 188 kcal, 0.49 g Fat, 8.37 g Total Carbs, 6.98 g Protein, 5.5 g Fiber

Spinach & Lettuce Leaves Salad

Prep Time 15 Min

Servings 2

Ingredients:
- 1 pack baby spinach
- 1 red onion thinly sliced
- 1 pack lettuce leaves, chopped
- 2 oz. dry cherry tomatoes

DRESSING
- 1 tbsp. olive oil
- 1 tbsp. lime juice
- 1 pinch salt and pepper

Directions:
1. Cut veggies and pour in a mixing bowl; mix thoroughly.
2. Mix dressing ingredients in the bowl and pour over veggies.
3. Serve cold and enjoy!

Nutritional information:
Calories Per Servings, 237 kcal, 15.49 g Fat, 15.49 g Total Carbs, 7.3 g Protein, 9.7 g Fiber

Tofu Salad with Spinach

Prep Time 15 Min

Servings 2

Ingredients:
- 1 pack baby spinach
- 1/2 avocado, chopped
- 1 red onion, chopped.
- ½ cup tofu
- 1 tbsp. sesame oil
- 1 lime juice
- 1 pinch garlic salt

Directions:
1. Mash and mix all veggies in a mixing bowl with tofu.
2. Add in oil, lime juice, and garlic salt.
3. Serve cold and enjoy!

Nutritional information:
Calories Per Servings, 121 kcal, 0.49 g Fat, 32.2 g Total Carbs, 0.85 g Protein, 5.3 g Fiber

Tofu & Berries Salad

Prep Time 15 Min

Servings 2

Ingredients:
- 1 pack arugula leaves
- 8 oz. strawberries, sliced
- 1 oz. walnuts
- 2 oz. smoked tofu

Dressing
- 1 tbsp. olive oil
- 1 lime juice
- 1 pinch garlic salt

Directions:
1. Put all veggies in a mixing bowl and mix thoroughly.
2. Mix dressing ingredients in the bowl and pour over veggies.
3. Serve cold and enjoy!

Nutritional information:
Calories Per Servings, 271 kcal, 22.09 g Fat, 15.48 g Total Carbs, 7.89 g Protein, 4.4 g Fiber

Pomegranate & Spinach Salad

Prep Time 15 Min

Servings 2

Ingredients:
- 1 pack baby spinach
- 1 cup pomegranate seeds
- 4-5 lettuce leaves, chopped

Dressing
- 1 tbsp. olive oil
- 1 lime juice
- 1 pinch garlic salt

Directions:
1. Put all veggies in a mixing bowl and mix thoroughly.
2. Mix dressing ingredients in the bowl and pour over veggies.
3. Serve cold and enjoy!

Nutritional information:
Calories Per Servings, 237 kcal, 9.35 g Fat, 37.15 g Total Carbs, 8.89 g Protein, 10.8 g Fiber

Olives & Green Salad

Prep Time 15 Min

Servings 2

Ingredients:
- 4-5 lettuce leaves
- 1 cucumber, sliced
- 1 red onion, cut into rings
- 1 tomato, sliced

Dressing
- 1 tbsp. olive oil
- 1 lime juice
- 1 pinch garlic salt
- I pinch pepper

Directions:
1. Put all veggies in a mixing bowl and mix thoroughly.
2. Mix dressing ingredients in the bowl and pour over veggies.
3. Lay lettuce leaves on a serving plate. Top with veggies.
4. Serve cold and enjoy!

Nutritional information: Calories Per Servings, 237 kcal, 9.35 g Fat, 37.15 g Total Carbs, 8.89 g Protein, 10.8 g Fiber

Green Salad with Tofu

Prep Time 15 Min

Servings 2

Ingredients:
- 1 pack baby spinach
- 1 cucumber, roughly sliced
- 2 oz. tofu crumbled
- I tomato, slice
- 4-5 lettuce leaves, chopped

Dressing
- 1 tbsp. olive oil
- 1 lime juice
- 1 pinch garlic salt

Directions:
1. Put all veggies in a mixing bowl and mix thoroughly.
2. Mix dressing ingredients in the bowl and pour over veggies.
3. Serve cold and enjoy!

Nutritional information:
Calories Per Servings, 237 kcal, 9.35 g Fat, 37.15 g Total Carbs, 8.89 g Protein, 10.8 g Fiber

Arugula & Chicken Salad

Prep Time 15 Min

Servings 2

Ingredients:
- 1 pack arugula leaves
- 2 oz. grilled chicken steak, sliced
- 1 Tomato, sliced

Dressing
- 1 tbsp. olive oil
- 1 lime juice
- 1 pinch garlic salt

Directions:
1. Put all veggies and chicken in a mixing bowl and mix thoroughly.
2. Mix dressing ingredients in a bowl and pour over veggies.
3. Serve cold and enjoy!

Green Juicy Salad Bowl

Prep Time 10 min

Servings 2

Ingredients:
- 1 bag, baby spinach
- 1 cucumber, sliced
- 16 oz. broccoli, florets
- 1 bunch lettuce leaves
- 4 oz. tofu, fried.
- 2-3 tomatoes, sliced

DRESSING
- 2 tbsps. raw apple cider vinegar
- 1 tbsp. olive
- 2 garlic cloves, minced
- 2 tbsps. lemon juice
- 1 tsp dijon mustard
- 1/4 tsp salt
- 2 tbsps. water optional

Directions:
1. Mix dressing ingredients in a bowl and set aside.
2. Fry tofu in pan until brown.
3. Steam broccoli in a microwave with some water.

4. Chop veggies and arrange in the bowl with tofu and broccoli.
5. Drizzle dressing over veggies.
6. Slightly mix.
7. Serve and enjoy!

Nutritional information:
Calories Per Servings, 229 kcal, 13.26 g Fat, 17.61 g Protein, 17.93 g Total Carbs, 9 g Fiber

Green Salad with Flaxseed

Prep Time 15 Min

Servings 2

Ingredients:
- 1 pack arugula leaves
- 1 cucumber sliced
- 1 red bell pepper, sliced
- 2-3 tomatoes, sliced
- 1 tsp. flaxseeds

Dressing
- 1 tbsp. Italian seasoning
- 1 tbsp. olive oil
- 4 tbsps. red wine vinegar
- ½ tsp salt
- ¼ tsp ground black pepper
- 1 tbsp. Dijon mustard

Directions:
1. Put all veggies in a mixing bowl and mix thoroughly.
2. Mix dressing ingredients in a bowl and pour over veggies.
3. Serve cold and enjoy!

Nutritional information:
Calories Per Servings, 110 kcal, 8.08 g Fat, 2.29 g Protein, 7.86 g Total Carbs, 2.5 g Fiber

Green Salad with Spinach

Prep Time 15 Min

Servings 2

Ingredients:
- 1 pack lettuce leaves, chopped
- 1 cucumber, sliced
- 8 oz. strawberries, sliced
- 1 tsp. flaxseeds

Dressing
- 1 tbsp. olive oil
- 3/4 cup apple cider vinegar
- 1/4 cup prepared mustard
- 1 tbsp. soy sauce
- 1 tbsp. Splenda
- 4 cloves garlic, minced
- 1 tsp. kosher salt
- 1 tsp. ground black pepper

Directions:
1. Cup and slice all veggies and arrange in serving plate.
2. Mix dressing ingredients in a bowl and pour over veggies.
3. Drizzle flax seeds on top.
4. Serve cold and enjoy!

Nutritional information:
Calories Per Servings, 183 kcal, 10.41 g Fat, 3.61 g Protein, 17.66 g Total Carbs, 5 g Fiber

Tabbouleh with Lime Dressing

Prep Time 15 Min

Servings 2

Ingredients:
- 1 cucumber, finely chopped
- 8 oz. spinach, finely chopped
- 1 red onion finely chopped
- 1 cup buckwheat groats, cooked
- 8 oz. parsley, finely chopped
- 8 oz. strawberries, chopped

Dressing
- 3 cloves garlic, finely minced
- 1 ½ tsps. anchovy paste
- 1 tsp. Worcestershire sauce
- 2 tbsps. fresh lemon juice
- 1 ½ tsps. Dijon mustard
- Salt and Pepper to taste

Directions:
1. Put all chopped veggies and buckwheat in a mixing bowl and mix well.
2. Mix dressing ingredients in a bowl and pour over veggies.
3. Serve cold and enjoy!

Nutritional information:
Calories Per Servings, 238 kcal, 2.84 g Fat, 12.96 g Protein, 49.7 g Total Carbs, 12.1 g Fiber

Zucchini Olives And Beans Salad

Prep Time 10 Min
Cooking Time 25 min
Total Time 35 Min

Servings 4

Ingredients:
- 1 zucchini, thinly sliced
- 4 oz. black olives
- 1 cup white beans, cooked
- 1 cup cauliflower, steamed

- Salt and pepper
- 3–4 tbsps. lime juice
- 3–4 tbsps. olive oil

Directions:
1. Mix all ingredients in the serving platter.
2. Season with salt and pepper, and mix well.
3. Drizzle lime juice and oil on top.
4. Enjoy!

Nutritional information:
Calories Per Servings, 238 kcal, 2.84 g Fat, 12.96 g Protein, 49.7 g Total Carbs, 12.1 g Fiber

Salmon Mushrooms and Lentils

Prep Time 10 Min
Cooking Time 25 min
Total Time 35 Min
Servings 4

Ingredients:
- 8 oz. button mushrooms, sliced
- 8 oz. salmon steak, cut into slice
- 4 tomatoes, halves
- 1 cup red lentils cooked
- 4-6 lettuce leaves
- Sesame seeds
- 1 tbsps. olive oil
- salt & pepper

Directions:
1. Heat oil in pan over medium heat.
2. Once oil is hot, add salmon slice and cook for 2-3 minutes per side until cooked through.
3. Transfer cooked salmon in plate.
4. Pour sliced mushrooms in the same pan and cook for 4-5 minutes until cooked and shrink.
5. Pour salmon, mushrooms, tomatoes, lentils, lettuce leaves in a serving bowl.
6. Drizzle salt, pepper, and sesame seeds on top.
7. Serve and enjoy!

Nutritional information:
Calories Per Servings, 238 kcal, 2.84 g Fat, 12.96 g Protein, 49.7 g Total Carbs, 12.1 g Fiber

Onion & Avocado Salad

Prep Time 20 Min
Total Time 20 Min
Servings 2

Ingredients:
- 1 avocado, thinly sliced
- 1 red onion, thinly sliced
- 1 bunch lettuce leaves, chopped

Directions:
1. Spread out chopped lettuce leaves on a platter.
2. Top with an avocado slice and red onion slice.
3. Serve and enjoy!

Nutritional information:
Calories Per Servings, 238 kcal, 2.84 g Fat, 12.96 g Protein, 49.7 g Total Carbs, 12.1 g Fiber

Tuna & Veggies Salad

Prep Time 15 Min
Total Time 15 Min
Servings 2

Ingredients:
- 1 egg, boil cut into halves
- 1 cup tuna, steamed
- 1 red onion sliced
- 1 avocado sliced.
- 4-5 cherry tomato, sliced
- 4-5 lettuce leaves, chopped
- 4 oz. green beans
- 1 lemon, halves
- Salt and pepper to taste
- 6 tbsps. lemon juice

Directions:
1. Boil an egg in salted water for about 4-6 minutes.
2. Steam tuna for about 4-5 minutes.
3. For serving add tuna, egg, tomatoes, beans, lettuce leaves in a bowl.
4. Drizzle salt, pepper, and lemon juice on top.
5. Serve and enjoy!

Nutritional information:
Calories Per Servings, 238 kcal, 2.84 g Fat, 12.96 g Protein, 49.7 g Total Carbs, 12.1 g Fiber

Watermelon & Raspberry Salad

Prep Time 15 Min
Total Time 15 Min
Servings 2

Ingredients:
- 4 cups watermelon, cut
- 1 cup raspberries
- 1 cup crumble feta cheese
- 5-10 fresh mint leaves

Directions:
1. Cut watermelon into cubes and pour in serving bowls.
2. Top with raspberries, feta cheese, and mint leaves.
3. Serve chill and enjoy it!

Greek Salad with Olives

Prep Time 15 Min
Total Time 15 Min

Servings 2

Ingredients:

- 4 oz. olives
- 4 oz. feta cheese, cubes
- 1 cucumber sliced
- 2-3 red tomatoes slices
- 2-3 yellow tomatoes, sliced
- red onion sliced
- 1 cup spinach, finely chopped
- 1/4 lemon juice
- 4-5 tbsps. olive oil
- salt & pepper

Directions:

1. Cut and chopped vegetables and mix in a bowl.
2. Pour lemon juice, olive oil, salt, and pepper, and mix well.
3. Serve chill and enjoy it!

Salmon With Veggies

Prep Time 10 Min
Cooking Time 20 min
Total Time 30 Min

Servings: 2

Ingredients:

- 1 salmon steak cut into cubes.
- ½ cup lemon juice
- 1 tbsp. black pepper
- ½ tsp salt
- 2 tbsps. olive oil
- 2-4 tomatoes, sliced
- 4-5 lettuce leaves
- 1 lemon, cut into 4 pieces
- 1 tsp. sesame seeds

Directions:

1. Heat the oil in a pan over medium heat.
2. Once the oil is hot, add salmon and cook for 4-5 minutes. until cooked.
3. Cut vegetables and assemble in a serving bowl.
4. Top with salmon bites.
5. season with salt and pepper, and mix well.
6. Drizzle lime juice, olive oil, and sesame seeds on top.
7. Serve and enjoy!

Lettuce Salad & Grilled Prawns

Prep Time 10 Min
Cooking Time 20 min
Total Time 30 Min

Servings 4

Ingredients:

- 1 lb. peeled and deveined shrimp
- 2 tsps. taco seasoning
- 2 tbsps. olive oil
- lettuce leaves
- tomatoes
- lime juice

Directions:

1. Heat the oil in a pan over medium heat.
2. Once the oil is hot, add shrimp and cook for 4-5 minutes. until cooked.
3. Cut vegetables and assemble in a serving bowl.
4. Top with shrimp and season with salt and pepper, and mix well.
5. Drizzle lime juice, olive oil on top.
6. Serve and enjoy!

Main Meal Recipes

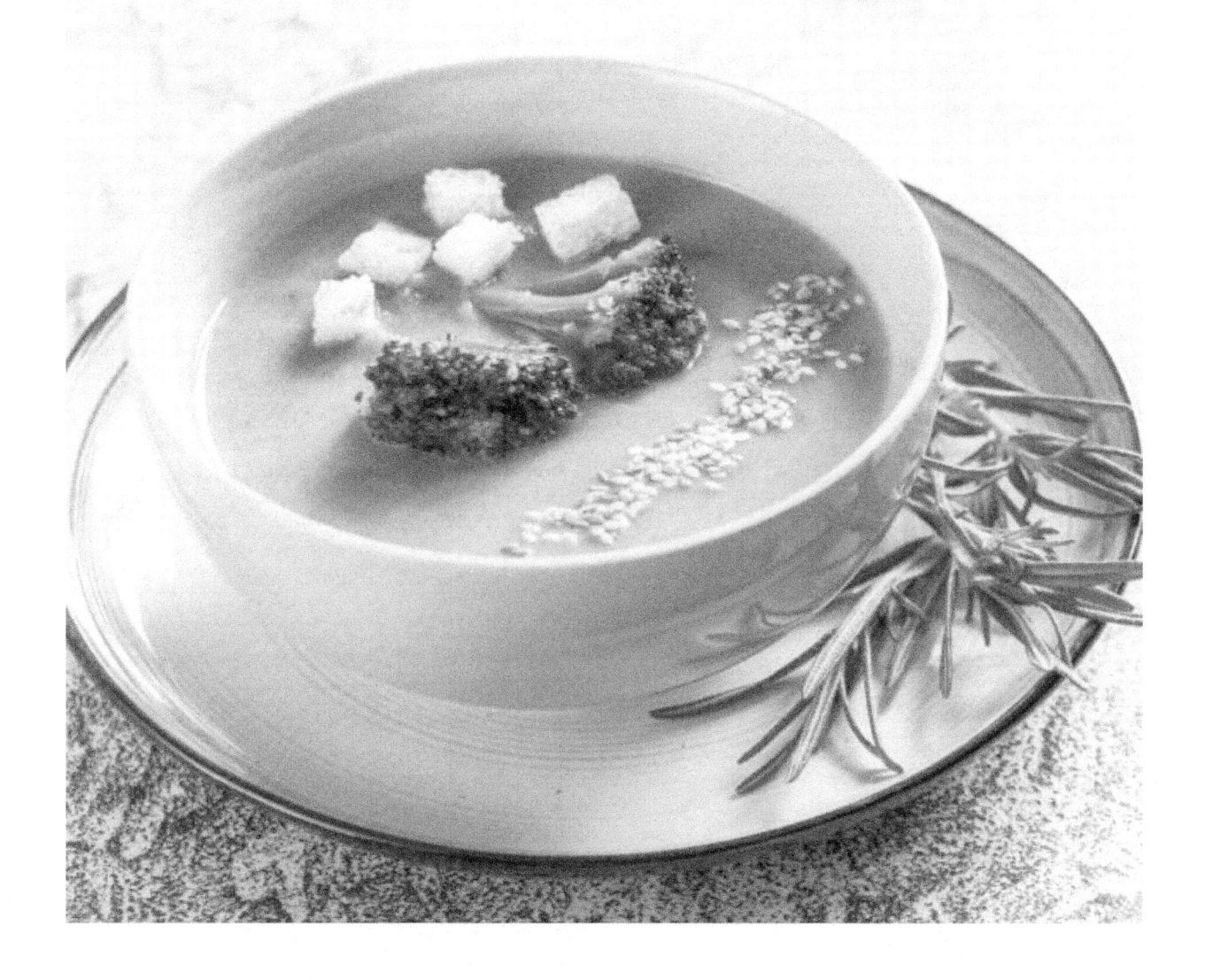

Creamy Spinach Curry

Prep Time 20 Min

Servings 4

Ingredients:
- 1 lb. spinach, chopped
- 1 tsp. ginger garlic paste
- salt & pepper to taste
- 1 tsp. paprika powder
- 1 tsp. cumin seeds
- 1 tsp red chili powder
- 1/2 tsp. turmeric powder
- 1 tbsp. olive oil
- ½ cup walnut cream

Directions:
1. Heat the oil in a pan over medium heat.
2. Once the oil is hot, add ginger garlic paste and cook for a minute.
3. Add chopped spinach in pan and cook for 4-5 minutes until spinach is welted.
4. Add rest of the spices and mix well.
5. Blender spinach in blender for 1 minute.
6. Pour spinach in a pan again, add walnut cream and cook on low heat for about 4-5 minutes.
7. Once cooked remove from heat, drizzle cream on top.
8. Enjoy!

Nutritional information:
Calories Per Servings, 125 kcal, 9.84 g Fat, 4.51 g Protein, 7.47 g Total Carbs, 3.1 g Fiber

Broccoli Olives Pizza

Prep Time 30 min

Servings 8

Ingredients:
- 1 lb. buckwheat pizza dough
- 2 tbsp. olive oil
- 1 bunch broccoli, cut into florets.
- 1 red onion, sliced
- 1 tsp minced garlic
- salt & pepper to taste
- 1 oz. BBQ sauce
- 2 oz. olives
- 6 oz. tofu, sliced

Directions:
1. Heat oil in skillet over medium heat.
2. Once the oil is hot, sauté onion and garlic for 2-3 minutes.
3. Season with spices and mix well.
4. Add broccoli in skillet and cook for about 5 minutes.
5. Preheat oven to 400.
6. Set buckwheat pizza dough over greased pizza pan.
7. Cover dough with BBQ sauce. Layer with tofu sliced, cooked broccoli, and broccoli.
8. Bake for about 10 minutes.
9. Serve hot and enjoy!

Nutritional information:
Calories Per Servings, 296 kcal, 10.7 g Fat, 11.44 g Protein, 44.03 g Total Carbs, 6.9 g Fiber

Buffalo Broccoli Bites

Prep Time 40 min

Servings 4

Ingredients:
- 1 head of broccoli, cut into bite-sized florets
- 1 cup buckwheat flour
- 3/4 cup soy milk
- 2 tsps. garlic powder
- 1 1/2 tsps. paprika powder
- salt &black pepper
- 1 tsp. oregano
- 3/4 cup breadcrumbs
- 1 cup spicy BBQ sauce

Directions:
1. Mix flour, soy milk, water, garlic powder, paprika powder, salt, and black pepper in a mixing bowl.
2. Dip the florets into the batter until they are coated well.
3. Roll florets over the breadcrumbs.
4. Arrange the florets over a baking tray and bake for 25 minutes at 350 °F.
5. Transfer the cooked broccoli bits to a bowl and coat BBQ sauce over it and bake again for 20 minutes at 350 °F.
6. Serve immediately and enjoy!

Nutritional information:
Calories Per Servings, 161 kcal, 2.77 g Fat, 7.62 g Protein, 30.1 g Total Carbs, 5.5 g Fiber

Spinach Soup

Prep Time 20 Min

Servings 4

Ingredients:
- 1 lb. spinach, chopped
- 1 tsp. ginger garlic paste
- salt & pepper to taste
- 1 tsp. paprika powder
- 1 tsp. cumin seeds
- 1 tsp red chili powder
- 1/2 tsp. turmeric powder
- 1 tbsp. olive oil
- 3 cups vegetable broth

Directions:
1. Heat the oil in a pan over medium heat.
2. Once the oil is hot, add ginger garlic paste and cook for a minute.
3. Add chopped spinach in pan and cook for 4-5 minutes until spinach is welted.
4. Add rest of the spices and mix well.
5. Blender spinach in blender for 1 minute.
6. Pour spinach in a pan again, add broth and cook on low heat for about 4-5 minutes.
7. Once cooked remove from heat, drizzle cream on top.
8. Enjoy

Nutritional information:
Calories Per Servings, 67 kcal, 4.05 g Fat, 3.7 g Protein, 6.37 g Total Carbs, 3.1 g Fiber

Chili Tofu

Prep Time 20 Min

Servings 4

Ingredients:
- 8 oz. tofu cut into cubes
- 1 tbsp. extra-virgin olive oil
- 2 large garlic cloves, minced
- 1 tsp. chili flakes
- salt & pepper
- 1 red chili, cut into rings
- 2 tbsps. green onion
- Salt and freshly ground black pepper

Directions:
1. Heat a large heavy skillet over medium heat. Add the oil, once the oil is hot, add the tofu with garlic cook for 5-8 minutes until brown.
2. Season with spices and add red chili rings.
3. Drizzle green onion on top.
4. Serve and enjoy!

Nutritional information:
Calories Per Servings, 174 kcal, 12.99 g Fat, 10.02 g Protein, 7.56 g Total Carbs, 2.5 g Fiber

Spicy Spinach Fillet

Prep Time 20 min

Servings 4

Ingredients:
- 1 cup buckwheat Flour
- 2 cups spinach, chopped
- 1/2 cup Onions, chopped
- 1 tsp. red chill
- 1/2 cup Kale, chopped
- 2 tsp. Basil
- 2 tsp. Oregano
- ½ cup water
- Olive Oil for frying

Directions:
1. Mix all seasonings and vegetables in a large bowl.
2. Add flour and spicy in the same bowl with seasoning and mix.
3. Add water to this mixture and mix.
4. The mixture should be thick enough to make patties.
5. Heat oil in skillet over medium heat.
6. Once the oil is hot, cook patties in skillet for about 2-3 minutes.
7. Flip and cook for another 2-3 minutes until both sides are brown.
8. Serve with tomato slices and enjoy.

Nutritional information:
Calories Per Servings, 119 kcal, 1.07 g Fat, 4.75 g Protein, 25.11 g Total Carbs, 4.1 g Fiber

Broccoli Patties

Prep Time 20 min

Servings 4

Ingredients:
- 1 cup buckwheat Flour
- 1 cup broccoli, chopped
- 1/2 cup Onions, chopped
- 1/2 cup Green Peppers, chopped
- 1/2 cup Kale, chopped
- 2 tsp. Basil
- 2 tsp. Oregano
- 2 tsp. Onion Powder
- 1/2 tsp. Ginger Powder
- ½ cup water
- Olive Oil for frying

Directions:
1. Mix all seasonings and vegetables in a large bowl.
2. Add flour and broccoli in the same bowl with seasoning and mix thoroughly.
3. Add water to this mixture and mix.
4. The mixture should be thick enough to make patties.
5. Heat oil in skillet over medium heat.
6. Once the oil is hot, cook patties in skillet for about 2-3 minutes.
7. Flip and cook for another 2-3 minutes until both sides are brown.
8. Serve hot and enjoy!

Nutritional information:
Calories Per Servings, 117 kcal, 1.06 g Fat, 4.63 g Protein, 24.85 g Total Carbs, 4.1 g Fiber

Spinach & Tofu Pizza

Prep Time 40 Min

Servings 8

Ingredients:
- 1/2 lb. spinach, trimmed
- 1 lb. buckwheat pizza dough.
- 16 oz. tofu, cut into cubes
- salt & pepper to taste
- 1 tsp oregano
- 1 tsp. chili powder
- 1 tbsp. olive oil
- 1 oz. walnut cream

Directions:
1. Preheat the oven to 400°F.
2. Sautee spinach in a skillet over medium heat, for about 10 minutes until spinach is wilted.
3. Season with spices and mix well.
4. Set pizza dough over greased pizza pan.
5. Spread the walnut cream over pizza dough then spread spinach.
6. Top with tofu bites.
7. Bake pizza for about 20 minutes in preheated oven.
8. Once cooked remove from oven.
9. Serve and enjoy.

Nutritional information:
Calories Per Servings, 254 kcal, 15.93 g Fat, 13.17 g Protein, 19.63 g Total Carbs, 4.8 g Fiber

Broccoli Flatbread Pizza

Prep Time 30 min

Servings 8

Ingredients:
- 1 lb. buckwheat dough
- 2 tbsp. olive oil
- 1 bunch broccoli, cut into florets.
- 1 red onion, sliced
- 1 tsp minced garlic
- salt & pepper to taste
- 1 oz. walnut cream

Directions:
1. Heat oil in skillet over medium heat.
2. Once the oil is hot, sauté onion and garlic for 2-3 minutes.
3. Season with spices and mix well.
4. Add broccoli in skillet and cook for about 5 minutes.
5. Preheat oven to 400.
6. Set buckwheat dough over greased pizza pan.
7. Cover dough with walnut cream. Layer with cooked broccoli.
8. Bake for about 10 minutes.
9. Serve hot and enjoy!

Nutritional information:
Calories Per Servings, 112 kcal, 6.13 g Fat, 3.08 g Protein, 12.97 g Total Carbs, 2.3 g Fiber

Turmeric Spinach Patties

Prep Time 20 min

Servings 4

Ingredients:
- 1 cup buckwheat Flour
- 2 cups spinach, chopped
- 1/2 cup Onions, chopped
- 1 tbsp. turmeric
- 1/2 cup Kale, chopped
- 2 tsp. Basil
- 2 tsp. Oregano
- 2 tsp. Onion Powder
- 1/2 tsp. Ginger Powder
- ½ cup spring water
- Olive oil for frying

Directions:
1. Mix all seasonings and vegetables in a large bowl.
2. Add flour and spinach in the same bowl with seasoning and mix thoroughly.
3. Add water to this mixture and mix.
4. The mixture should be thick enough to make patties.
5. Heat oil in skillet over medium heat.
6. Once the oil is hot, cook patties in skillet for about 2-3 minutes. Flip and cook for another 2-3 minutes until both sides are brown.
7. Serve hot and enjoy!

Nutritional information:
Calories Per Servings, 124 kcal, 1.13 g Fat, 4.86 g Protein, 26.16 g Total Carbs, 4.6 g Fiber

Stir Fried Broccoli & Tofu

Prep Time 20 Min

Servings 4

Ingredients:
- 8 oz. tofu cut into cubes
- 16 oz. broccoli cut into
- 1 tbsp. extra-virgin olive oil
- 2 large garlic cloves, minced
- Salt and freshly ground black pepper
- 2 oz. walnut cream
- Spinach leaves

Directions:
1. Heat a large heavy skillet over medium heat. Add the oil, once the oil is hot, add broccoli with garlic and cook for 4-8 minutes until cooked.
2. Transfer cooked broccoli to a plate.
3. Add the tofu cook for another 5-8 minutes until brown.
4. Transfer cooked tofu with broccoli and assemble spinach with them.
5. Drizzle walnut cream, salt, and pepper on top.
6. Serve and enjoy!

Nutritional information:
Calories Per Servings, 287 kcal, 22.75 g Fat, 15.81 g Protein, 11.62 g Total Carbs, 6.3 g Fiber

Wilted Spinach with Onion

Prep Time 40 Min

Servings 2

Ingredients:
- 4 red onions, cut into rings
- 1/4 cup olive oil
- 2 1lb. spinach with stems
- Salt and freshly ground pepper

Directions:
1. Heat oil in a large pan over medium heat.
2. Add the onion rings and cook for about 10-15 minutes over low heat until the onion is caramelized.
3. Transfer onion to plate.
4. Add spinach in the same pan and cook for about 5-10 minutes until about to wilted.
5. Transfer spinach to plate.
6. Top with caramelized onion.
7. Drizzle salt & pepper on top.
8. Serve and enjoy!

Nutritional information:
Calories Per Servings, 300 kcal, 22.79 g Fat, 13.6 g Protein, 18.13 g Total Carbs, 11.1 g Fiber

Broccoli with Garlic sauce

Prep Time 30 Min

Servings 2

Ingredients:
- 1/3 cup minced fresh garlic
- 2 tablespoons olive oil
- 1 head broccoli cut into florets with stems
- 1 cup vegetable broth
- 1 tsp. turmeric
- salt & pepper to taste
- 1 tbsp. buckwheat flour

Directions:
1. Heat oil in skillet over medium he
2. Add broccoli florets and cook for 4-5 minutes. Set aside.
3. Add minced garlic in the same skillet and cook for 3 - 5 minutes, until garlic begins to brown.
4. Add broth salt & pepper and flour and mix well.
5. Pour broccoli in skillet again and cook for another 4-5 minutes until broccoli is soft and sauce is thick.
6. Serve hot and enjoy!

Nutritional information:
Calories Per Servings, 282 kcal, 14.95 g Fat, 11.07 g Protein, 33.39 g Total Carbs, 9.4 g Fiber

Hot & Sour Spinach

Prep Time 40 Min

Servings 2

Ingredients:
- 1 red onion, minced
- 1/2 cup sherry vinegar
- 1 thyme sprig
- 1 tablespoon dates syrup
- 2 1lb. spinach
- 3 tablespoons extra-virgin olive oil
- Salt and freshly ground pepper
- 1 cup vegetable broth

Directions:
1. Heat oil in pan over medium heat.
2. Add the onion and cook for about 2-3 minutes over low heat.
3. Add the vinegar and thyme sprig and bring to a boil.
4. Simmer over low heat until the vinegar is reduced.
5. Add dates syrup and mix well.
6. Add broth in pan, bring to a boil.
7. Add the spinach and cook until wilted.
8. Season with salt and pepper and cook for about 5 minutes.
9. Transfer the spinach to a platter with some broth.
10. Serve and enjoy!

Nutritional information:
Calories Per Servings, 296 kcal, 11.86 g Fat, 15.79 g Protein, 37.91 g Total Carbs, 12.3 g Fiber

Spinach & Tofu Curry

Prep Time 30 Min

Servings 4

Ingredients:
- 2 cups, tofu cubes
- 2 cups spinach, chopped
- 2 cloves

- 1 cardamom
- 2 tbsps. olive oil
- 1 green chili, chopped
- 1 onion, chopped
- 1 cup walnut milk
- ½ tsp. ginger-garlic paste
- 1 tsp. cumin seeds
- Salt to taste

Directions:
1. Heat oil in a pan over medium heat. once oil is hot, add tofu cubes and cook for 2-3 minutes.
2. Transfer fried tofu in plate.
3. Add the clove, cardamom, cinnamon, and cumin seeds and onion in pan and cook for 2-3 minutes.
4. Add spinach, milk, salt, and ginger-garlic paste.
5. Stir-fry for 10-15 minutes over medium heat
6. Add fried tofu stir and combine well.
7. Once cooked remove from heat.
8. Serve and enjoy!

Nutritional information:
Calories Per Servings, 237 kcal, 11.31 g Fat, 7.34 g Protein, 27.12 g Total Carbs, 1.1 g Fiber

Sardine Puttanesca Spaghetti

Prep Time 10 Min

Servings 4

Ingredients:
- 300-400 g buckwheat spaghetti
- 1 tbsp olive
- 2 garlic cloves, minced
- 1/4 tsp chill flakes, optional
- 2 tin chopped tomatoes
- 1 tin sardines in olive oil
- 2 tbsp pitted black olives, sliced
- 1 tbsp capers
- 2 cups frozen chopped kale
- handful of fresh parsley or chives, roughly chopped

Directions:
1. Bring a large pan of water to the boil and add a generous pinch of salt. When the water is boiling, add the spaghetti and simmer for 8-10 mins until al dente while you make the sauce.
2. Heat the oil in a large frying pan and add the garlic and chili flakes.
3. Cook for 30 secs-1 min then add the chopped tomatoes.
4. Cook for a couple of mins, then add the sardines, olives, capers, and kale.
5. Cook for another 4-5 mins, until sauce is cooked, sardines are broken up in the sauce and everything is heated through.
6. Drain the spaghetti and stir the sauce through it, then serve with the fresh herbs.

Nutritional information:
Calories Per Servings, 237 kcal, 11.31 g Fat, 7.34 g Protein, 27.12 g Total Carbs, 1.1 g Fiber

Tofu Power Bowls

Prep Time 50 Min

Servings 4

Ingredients:
- 1 cup buckwheat groats
- 1 package extra-firm tofu
- 1/2 tablespoons cornstarch
- 1 1/2 teaspoons chili powder
- 1 teaspoon kosher salt
- 1/2 teaspoon freshly ground black pepper
- 1/2 teaspoon garlic powder
- 2 teaspoons olive oil
- 2 cups shredded kale
- 1 1/2 cups shelled cooked edamame
- 2 carrots, peeled and grated
- 3/4 cup packed fresh cilantro leaves
- 1 lime, cut into wedges

For the creamy walnut sauce
- 1/4 cup creamy walnut butter
- 1 tablespoon reduced sodium soy sauce
- 1 tablespoon freshly squeezed lime juice
- 2 teaspoons dark brown sugar
- 1 teaspoon sambal oelek
- 1 teaspoon freshly grated ginger

Directions:
1. To make the walnut sauce, mix walnut butter, soy sauce, lime juice, brown sugar, sambal oelek, ginger, and 2-3 tablespoons water in a small bowl and set aside.
2. Cook buckwheat in water and cook for few minutes.
3. Preheat oven to 400 degrees F. Line a baking sheet with parchment paper.
4. In a large bowl mix crumbled tofu, cornstarch, chili powder, salt, pepper, and garlic powder. Stir in 1 tablespoon olive oil until well combined.
5. Bake tofu for 30 minutes, until golden brown and crispy.
6. In a small bowl, add kale and drizzle with the remaining 2 teaspoons olive oil; season with salt and pepper to taste. Massage until the kale starts to soften and wilt, about 1-2 minutes.
7. Divide buckwheat into bowls.
8. Top with tofu, kale, edamame, carrots, and cilantro.
9. Serve with creamy walnut sauce.
10. Enjoy!

Nutritional information:
Calories Per Servings, 237 kcal, 11.31 g Fat, 7.34 g Protein, 27.12 g Total Carbs, 1.1 g Fiber

Superfood Bibimbap With Crispy Tofu

Prep Time 45 Min

Servings 4

Ingredients:
- 1 block organic extra firm tofu, sliced
- 1/2 cup low sodium soy sauce
- 1-2 tablespoons chili paste
- tablespoons toasted sesame oil
- 1-inch fresh ginger, grated
- cloves garlic, grated
- 2 tablespoons extra virgin olive oil
- cup shiitake mushrooms, sliced or torn
- 1 bunch curly kale, roughly torn
- juice from 1 lime
- kosher salt
- 2 cups cooked buckwheat
- 1 avocado, sliced
- 1 cup fresh or pickled carrots and radishes

Directions:
1. Preheat the oven to 400 degrees F. Line a baking sheet with parchment paper.
2. Slice into 1/4-inch-thick slices and add to a gallon size Ziplock bag.
3. In a small bowl, mix the 2-tablespoon water, the soy sauce, chili paste, sesame oil, ginger, and garlic. Add half the sauce to the tofu bag tossing gently to combine. Let it sit for 5-10 minutes.
4. Remove the tofu from the sauce and bake for 10 minutes. Flip and bake another 10-15 minutes, until the tofu is crisp.
5. Meanwhile, toss mushrooms with 1 tablespoon oil and a pinch of salt.
6. Add the veggies to the pan with the tofu.
7. In a bowl, massage the kale with the remaining 1 tablespoons olive oil, lime juice, and a pinch of salt.
8. Divide the grains among bowls. Add the tofu, kale, mushrooms, avocado, carrots, and radishes.
9. Enjoy!

Nutritional information:
Calories Per Servings, 237 kcal, 11.31 g Fat, 7.34 g Protein, 27.12 g Total Carbs, 1.1 g Fiber

Spicy Tofu Kale Wraps

Prep Time 20 Min

Servings 2

Ingredients:
- 3 tablespoons soy sauce
- 2 tablespoon sesame oil
- 1-3 teaspoons chili paste
- 2 teaspoons ginger
- 2 teaspoons sugar
- 2 teaspoon rice vinegar
- 2 cloves garlic, minced
- 2 tablespoon vegetable oil
- 1 (12-ounce) package firm tofu
- 1 red bell pepper, diced
- 2 cups chopped mushrooms
- Kale leaves, for serving

Directions:
1. In a small bowl, mix soy sauce, sesame oil, chili paste, ginger, sugar, rice vinegar, and garlic; set aside.
2. Heat vegetable oil in a skillet over medium heat.
3. Add tofu and sear until golden brown, about 2-3 minutes on each side. Transfer to a paper towel-lined plate.
4. Add mushrooms and bell pepper to skillet and cook, stirring frequently until tender, about 3-4 minutes.
5. Stir in soy sauce mixture and cook until sauce has reduced slightly, about 2-3 minutes.
6. To serve, spoon several tablespoons of the tofu mixture into the center of a kale leaf.
7. Serve and enjoy!

Nutritional information:
Calories Per Servings, 237 kcal, 11.31 g Fat, 7.34 g Protein, 27.12 g Total Carbs, 1.1 g Fiber

Tofu Burritos

Prep Time 35 Min

Servings 8

Ingredients:
- 8 Tortillas

For eggless egg salad
- 12 oz tofu extra firm
- 1/3 cup vegenaise
- tbsp yellow mustard
- 1/4 tsp cayenne pepper
- 1 tsp turmeric
- tbsp fresh parsley chopped
- 1 tbsp dill chopped
- tbsp fresh cilantro chopped
- green onions chopped
- 1 cup cherry tomatoes chopped
- 1 tbsp lime juice
- salt and pepper to taste
- 1/2 tsp salt or to taste
- 1/4 tsp pepper or to taste

Directions:
1. In a large bowl crumble up the tofu using your hands.
2. Add the remaining ingredients for the eggless egg salad and stir well.
3. Adjust seasoning with salt and pepper as necessary.
4. To assemble the burritos, top each tortilla with 1/2 cup of the eggless egg salad.
5. Roll up the burritos and wrap them in foil.
6. Refrigerate leftover burritos wrapped in foil for about 2 to 3 days.
7. You can also heat them a bit in the microwave before serving.

Nutritional information:
Calories Per Servings, 237 kcal, 11.31 g Fat, 7.34 g Protein, 27.12 g Total Carbs, 1.1 g Fiber

Asian Garlic Tofu

Prep Time 60 Min

Servings 2

Ingredients:
- 1 package super firm tofu
- 1/4 cup Hoisin sauce
- 2 tablespoons soy sauce
- 1 teaspoon sugar
- 1 teaspoon freshly grated ginger
- 2 cloves garlic, minced
- 1/4 teaspoon red pepper flakes
- 1 tablespoon olive oil
- 1 teaspoon sesame oil
- green onions for garnish
- rice for serving

Directions:
1. Remove tofu from packaging. Place about 4 paper towels on a plate. Set tofu on top of the plate and cover with more paper towels. Place a cast iron pan or something else that is heavy on top. Let it sit for 30 minutes.
2. In a medium bowl, stir together Hoisin sauce, soy sauce, sugar, ginger, garlic, and red pepper flakes.
3. Cut tofu into bite-sized pieces. Place in bowl with sauce and toss to coat. Let sit for 30 minutes.
4. Heat olive oil in a medium cast-iron pan over medium-high heat. Once really hot, add tofu. Once nicely seared on the bottom, flip over. Continue to cook until seared on the bottom.
5. Drizzle with sesame oil and remove from heat.
6. Sprinkle with green onions.
7. Enjoy!

Nutritional information:
Calories Per Servings, 237 kcal, 11.31 g Fat, 7.34 g Protein, 27.12 g Total Carbs, 1.1 g Fiber

Tofu Burritos Recipe 2

Prep Time 35 Min

Servings 8

Ingredients:
- 16 oz soft tofu cut into 1/2-inch cubes
- ¼ lb. ground pork
- 1/2 tbsp sesame oil
- 1/2 tbsp doubanjiang roughly chopped
- 1 tbsp chili oil
- 1 cup water
- 1 tbsp low sodium soy sauce
- 2 garlic cloves minced
- 1 tsp grated ginger
- 1 tsp sugar
- 1-1/2 tbsp water + 1 tbsp cornstarch
- 2 green scallions, finely sliced
- 1/2 tsp Sichuan peppercorn powder

Directions:
1. To make peppercorn powder, fry 1 heaping tbsp of peppercorns in a small skillet with about 1 tsp of oil (any kind). Toss peppercorn until the aroma of peppercorns comes out. Pat dry and let cool. Place in a spice grinder and grind to powder. Set aside.
2. Bring a large pot of water to boil. Slide in tofu. Cook for about 1 minute. Drain tofu and set aside.
3. In a large skillet, add the ground pork and sesame oil and cook until pork is cooked. Then add in the doubanjiang, garlic, ginger, chili oil. Cook for about 1 minute.
4. Add in 1 cup of water. Bring to a boil and slide in tofu. Stir in soy sauce and sugar. Taste and adjust seasoning as needed. You can add more soy sauce if you feel it isn't salty enough. If you feel it isn't spicy enough you can add more chili oil or more doubanjiang. Keep in mind that you will also be adding peppercorn powder at the end which will add to the spiciness. If it is too spicy, you can add a little more sugar. Cook until sauce is reduced.
5. In a small bowl add 2 1/2 tbsp water and 1 tbsp cornstarch. Stir until cornstarch is completely dissolved into water. Add to sauce and immediately stir so that the cornstarch slurry dissolves into the sauce and doesn't clump up. Cook about 30 more seconds or until sauce is thickened.
6. Turn off heat and sprinkle peppercorn powder and scallions over the dish. If desired, you can also drizzle with a little more chili oil.
7. Serve immediately with rice or rice substitute of your choice.

Nutritional information:
Calories Per Servings, 237 kcal, 11.31 g Fat, 7.34 g Protein, 27.12 g Total Carbs, 1.1 g Fiber

Hot & Sour Soup

Prep Time 20 Min

Servings 4

Ingredients:
- 6 cups chicken or vegetable broth
- 14-ounce package water-packed extra-firm tofu, drained
- 1 cup mushrooms, thinly sliced
- 1/2 cup bamboo shoots
- 1/3 cup rice wine vinegar
- 6 tablespoons low sodium soy sauce
- 2 teaspoons minced garlic
- 2 teaspoon Gourmet Ginger
- 1/2 teaspoon crushed red pepper flakes

Directions:
1. Chop tofu into cubes and set aside.
2. Mix broth, vinegar, soy sauce, garlic, ginger, and crushed red pepper flakes in a large pot and bring to a boil.
3. Add in tofu, mushrooms, and bamboo shoots and cook on heat to medium-low.
4. Cook 5-10 minutes longer.
5. Garnish with dried cilantro or chives and serve immediately.

Nutritional information:
Calories Per Servings, 237 kcal, 11.31 g Fat, 7.34 g Protein, 27.12 g Total Carbs, 1.1 g Fiber

Tofu & Avocado Spring Rolls

Prep Time 20 Min

Servings 4

Ingredients:

Walnut dipping sauce
- 1/2 cup creamy walnut butter
- 2/3 cup water
- 2 Tablespoons hoisin sauce
- splash of fish sauce (optional)
- 2 garlic cloves, minced
- 1 teaspoon sugar

Buckwheat noodles, cooked according to instructions on the package
- 1 pound firm tofu, sliced and then cut into strips
- 1 tbsp. olive oil
- 1/2 red pepper, sliced into strips
- 1 avocado, sliced
- 1/2 cucumber, cut into strips
- 1/4 purple cabbage, sliced
- Thai basil leaves
- rice paper rice paper

Directions:
1. Mix walnut sauce Ingredients in a small mixing bowl.
2. Cook the noodles according to the instructions on the bag or box of noodles. After cutting the tofu into strips, place on a dry, clean paper towel.
3. Heat the oil on medium to medium-high for 4 to 5 minutes. Cook the tofu for about 4 to 5 minutes on each side.
4. Place on a plate lined with clean paper towels.
5. One at a time, wet the rice paper and then place it on a round plate.
6. Allow the rice paper to sit for at least one minute.
7. Add noodles, tofu, red pepper, avocado, cucumber, cabbage, and a couple of basil leaves and roll it.
8. Serve with the walnut dipping sauce.

Nutritional information:
Calories Per Servings, 237 kcal, 11.31 g Fat, 7.34 g Protein, 27.12 g Total Carbs, 1.1 g Fiber

Simple Tofu Quiche

Prep Time 45 Min

Servings 8

Ingredients:

Crust
- 3 medium-large potatoes, grated and squeezed
- 2 Tbsp melted vegan butter
- 1/4 tsp sea salt and pepper

Filling
- 12.3 ounces extra-firm silken tofu
- 2 Tbsp nutritional yeast
- 3 Tbsp hummus
- Sea salt and black pepper (to taste)
- 3 cloves garlic (chopped)
- 2 medium leeks chopped
- 3/4 cup cherry tomatoes (halved)
- 1 cup chopped kale

Directions:
1. Preheat oven to 450 degrees F (232 C) and grease quiche pan with cooking spray.
2. Add potatoes to a pie dish and drizzle with melted vegan butter and 1/4 tsp each salt and pepper. Toss to coat, then use fingers to press into the pan and up the sides to form an even layer.
3. Bake for 25-30 minutes or until golden brown all over. Set aside.
4. Prep veggies and garlic and add to a baking sheet. Toss with 2 Tbsp olive oil and a healthy pinch of each salt and pepper and toss to coat.
5. Place in the oven and bake until soft and golden brown (a total of 20-30 minutes). Set aside and lower oven heat to 375 degrees F (190 C).

6. Add drained tofu to a food processor with nutritional yeast, hummus, and a heaping 1/4 tsp each sea salt and black pepper. Set aside.
7. Remove veggies from the oven, add to a mixing bowl, and top with the tofu mixture. Toss to coat, then add to the crust and spread into an even layer.
8. Bake quiche at 375 degrees F (190 C) for a total of 30–40 minutes
9. Serve and enjoy!

Nutritional information:
Calories Per Servings, 237 kcal, 11.31 g Fat, 7.34 g Protein, 27.12 g Total Carbs, 1.1 g Fiber

Barbecued Waffle Iron Tofu

Prep Time 10 Min

Servings 2

Ingredients:
- 7 - 8 ounces extra-firm tofu
- 3 tablespoons Ketchup or tomato sauce
- 1 teaspoon barbecue seasoning
- 1/2 teaspoon soy sauce or gluten-free tamari
- 1/4 teaspoon spicy brown mustard or other prepared mustard
- 1 pinch stevia

Directions:
1. Drain the tofu and cut it into 3-4 equally thick pieces lengthwise.
2. On a shallow plate, mix the ketchup or tomato sauce with the barbecue rub, soy sauce, and mustard.
3. Combine well and add stevia. Drag each piece of tofu through the sauce until it's coated on all sides.
4. Preheat your waffle iron on its highest setting. Once it is hot, place the tofu on the iron, distributing it equally. Gently close the waffle iron and set a timer for 4-5 minutes.
5. Brush waffles with extra barbecue sauce and serve alone or on sandwiches.

Nutritional information:
Calories Per Servings, 237 kcal, 11.31 g Fat, 7.34 g Protein, 27.12 g Total Carbs, 1.1 g Fiber

Cauliflower Mac 'n' Cheese

Prep Time 30 Min

Servings 8

Ingredients:
- 3 tbsp. olive oil, divided, plus more for baking dish
- lb. buckwheat pasta
- medium-sized head cauliflower, florets
- 4 cloves garlic, sliced
- large yellow onion, thinly sliced
- Kosher salt and freshly ground black pepper
- 8 oz. tofu crumbled
- 1/4 tsp. mustard powder
- Pinch cayenne pepper
- 1/2 cup panko breadcrumbs
- 1/2 cup kale leaves chopped

Directions:
1. Cook pasta according to package Directions:.
2. Heat 2 tablespoons oil in a large pot over medium heat. Add cauliflower, garlic, and onion. Season with salt. Cook, covered, stirring occasionally, until tender, 15 to 20 minutes. Add 4 cups water and simmer until vegetables are very soft, 10 to 12 minutes. Drain, reserving 2 cups cooking liquid; let cool slightly.
3. Mix vegetables, tofu, mustard powder, and cayenne in a blender.
4. Purée, adding just enough reserved cooking liquid to get the mixture moving, until smooth, 1 to 2 minutes.
5. Add sauce to pasta and toss to combine. Transfer to prepared baking dish. Toss together panko, kale, and the remaining tablespoon of oil in a bowl.
6. Season with salt and pepper. Sprinkle over pasta.
7. Serve and enjoy!

Nutritional information:
Calories Per Servings, 237 kcal, 11.31 g Fat, 7.34 g Protein, 27.12 g Total Carbs, 1.1 g Fiber

Beans & Broccolini

Prep Time 15 Min

Servings 4

Ingredients:
- Kosher salt and freshly ground black pepper
- 1 lb. Broccolini, trimmed
- tbsp. olive oil
- tsp. lemon zest, plus 2 tablespoons juice
- tbsp. capers, drained and chopped
- tbsp. honey mustard
- 1/2 red pepper flakes
- 1 (15.5-ounce) can small white beans, rinsed

Directions:
1. Boil Broccolini in salted water and cook until stalks are crisp-tender, 1 to 2 minutes.
2. Whisk together oil, lemon zest and juice, capers, mustard, and red pepper flakes in a bowl.
3. Season with salt and pepper.
4. Add Broccolini and beans; toss to coat.

Nutritional information:
Calories Per Servings, 237 kcal, 11.31 g Fat, 7.34 g Protein, 27.12 g Total Carbs, 1.1 g Fiber

Chicken Stew

Prep Time 20 Min

Servings 4

Ingredients:
- 2 tablespoons extra-virgin olive oil
- 1 yellow onion, chopped
- 1 tablespoon garlic, minced
- 1 tablespoon fresh ginger, minced
- 1 teaspoon ground turmeric
- 1 teaspoon ground cumin
- 1 teaspoon ground coriander
- 1 teaspoon paprika
- 4 (6-ounce) boneless, skinless chicken thighs, trimmed and cut into 1-inch pieces
- 4 tomatoes, chopped
- 14 oz. walnut milk
- Salt and ground black pepper, as required
- 6 cups fresh Swiss chard, chopped
- 2 tablespoons fresh lemon juice

Directions:
1. Heat olive oil in a large heavy-bottomed soup pan over medium heat and sauté the onion for about 3- 4 minutes.
2. Add the ginger, garlic, and spices, and sauté for about 1 minute.
3. Add the chicken and cook for about 4-5 minutes.
4. Add the tomatoes, coconut milk, salt, and black pepper, and bring to a gentle simmer.
5. Adjust the heat to low and simmer, covered for about 10-15 minutes.
6. Stir in the Swiss chard and cook for about 4-5 minutes.
7. Add in lemon juice and remove from the heat.
8. Serve hot.

Baked Chicken with Salad

Prep Time 40 Min

Servings 4

Ingredients:

For Chicken
- 4 boneless, skinless chicken breast halves
- Salt and ground black pepper, as required
- 2 tablespoons extra-virgin olive oil

For Salad
- 4 cups fresh kale, tough ribs removed and chopped
- 2 cups carrots, peeled and julienned
- ¼ cup walnuts

For Dressing
- 1 small garlic clove, minced
- 2 tablespoons fresh lime juice
- 2 tablespoons extra-virgin olive oil
- 1 teaspoon raw honey
- ½ teaspoon Dijon mustard
- Salt and ground black pepper, as required

Directions:
1. Season chicken breast half with salt and black pepper evenly.
2. Heat the oil in a 12-inch sauté pan over medium-low heat.
3. Place the chicken breast and cook for about 9-10 minutes, without moving.
4. Flip the chicken breasts and cook for about 6 minutes or until cooked through.
5. Remove the sauté pan from heat and let the chicken stand in the pan for about 3 minutes.
9. Transfer the chicken breasts onto a cutting board for about 5 minutes.
10. Place all ingredients in a salad bowl and mix.
11. Mix all ingredients in another bowl and beat until well combined.
12. Cut each chicken breast into desired-sized slices.
13. Place the salad onto each serving plate and top each with chicken slices.
14. Drizzle with dressing and serve.

Lamb Chops with Salad

Prep Time 40 Min

Servings 4

Ingredients:

For Lamb Chops
- 2 tablespoons extra-virgin olive oil, divided
- 4 garlic cloves, crushed
- 1 tablespoon fresh rosemary leaves, minced
- 1 tablespoon fresh parsley leaves, minced
- Salt and ground black pepper, as required
- 4 (8-ounce) (1¼-inch-thick) lamb loin chops

For salad
- 4 cups fresh kale, tough ribs removed and torn
- 2 oranges, peeled and segmented
- 2 grapefruits, peeled and segmented
- 4 tablespoons unsweetened dried cranberries
- ½ teaspoon white sesame seeds

For Dressing
- 3 tablespoons extra-virgin olive oil
- 3 tablespoons fresh orange juice
- 2 teaspoons Dijon mustard
- 1 teaspoon raw honey
- Salt and ground black pepper, as required

Directions:
1. In a large bowl, add 1 tablespoon extra-virgin olive oil, garlic, herbs, salt, and black pepper, and mix well.
2. Add the chops and coat with mixture generously.
3. Preheat oven to 400 degrees F.
4. cook the lamb chops for about 3 minutes per side in a heavy-bottomed skillet.
6. Bake chop in preheated oven for about 10 minutes.
7. Remove the lamb chops from the oven and place onto a platter.
8. Meanwhile, in a salad bowl, place all ingredients and mix.
9. Mix all ingredients in another bowl and beat until well combined.
10. Place dressing on top of salad and toss to coat well.
11. Divide the salad onto serving plates and top each with chops.
12. Serve immediately.

Flank Steak with Salad

Prep Time 40 Min

Servings 4

Ingredients:
For Steak
- 2 tablespoons extra-virgin olive oil
- 4 (6-ounce) flank steaks
- Salt and ground black pepper, as required

For Salad
- 6 cups fresh baby arugula
- 1 cup cherry tomatoes, halved
- 1 cup cucumber, chopped
- 3 tablespoons extra-virgin olive oil
- 2 tablespoons red wine vinegar
- Salt and ground black pepper, as required

Directions:
1. Heat oil over medium-high heat and cook the steaks with salt and black pepper for about 4-5 minutes per side or until desired doneness.
2. Meanwhile, put all salad in a bowl and mix well.
3. Divide the arugula salad onto serving plates and top each with 1 steak.
4. Serve immediately.

Glazed Flank Steak

Prep Time 40 Min

Servings 4

Ingredients:
- 2 tablespoons arrowroot flour
- Salt and ground black pepper, as required
- 1½ pounds flank steak, cut into ¼-inch thick slices
- ½ cup extra-virgin olive oil, divided
- 1 onion, sliced
- 2 garlic cloves, minced
- 1 teaspoon fresh ginger, minced
- ¼ teaspoon red pepper flakes, crushed
- 1/3 cup raw honey
- ½ cup homemade beef broth
- ½ cup low-sodium soy sauce
- 5 tablespoons cashews
- 2 tablespoons fresh parsley, chopped

Directions:
1. Mix arrowroot flour, salt, and black pepper in a bowl.
2. Coat the beef slices in arrowroot flour mixture evenly and then shake off excess mixture.
3. For sauce: In a pan, heat 1 tablespoon of oil over medium heat and sauté the onion for about 3-4 minutes.
4. Add garlic, ginger, and red pepper flakes and sauté for about 1 minute.
5. Add the honey, broth, and soy sauce and stir to combine well.
6. Increase the heat to high and cook for about 3 minutes, stirring continuously.
7. Remove the sauce from heat and set aside.
8. In a large sauté pan, heat the remaining oil over medium-high heat and fry the beef slices for about 3-4 minutes.
9. With a slotted spoon, transfer the beef slices onto a paper towel-lined plate to drain.
10. Remove the oil from the sauté pan, leaving about 1 tablespoon inside.
11. Return the beef slices into sauté pan over medium heat and sear the beef slices for about 2-3 minutes.
12. Stir in honey sauce and cook for about 3-5 minutes.
13. Serve hot with the garnishing of cashews and parsley.

Salmon & Lentils

Prep Time 40 Min

Servings 4

Ingredients:
For Lentils
- ½ pound French green lentils
- 2 tablespoons extra-virgin olive oil
- 2 cups yellow onions, chopped
- 2 cups scallions, chopped
- 1 teaspoon fresh parsley, chopped
- Salt and ground black pepper, as required
- 1 tablespoon fresh garlic, minced
- 1½ cups carrots, peeled and chopped
- 1½ cups celery stalks, chopped

- 1 tomato, crushed finely
- 1½ cups homemade chicken broth
- 2 tablespoons red wine vinegar

For Salmon
- 4 (6-ounce) skinless salmon fillets
- 2 tablespoons extra-virgin olive oil
- Salt and ground black pepper, as required

Directions:
1. In a heat-proof bowl, soak the lentils in boiling water for 15 minutes.
2. Drain the lentils completely.
3. In a Dutch oven, heat the oil over medium heat and cook the onions, scallions, parsley, salt, and black pepper for about 10 minutes, stirring frequently.
4. Add the garlic and cook for about 2 more minutes.
5. Add the drained lentils, carrots, celery, crushed tomato, and broth, and bring to a boil.
6. Reduce the heat to low and simmer, covered for about 20-25 minutes.
7. Stir in the vinegar, salt, and black pepper and remove from the heat.
8. Meanwhile, for salmon: Preheat the oven to 450 degrees F.
9. Rub the salmon fillets with oil and then, season with salt and black pepper generously.
10. Heat an oven-proof sauté pan over medium heat and cook the salmon fillets for about 2 minutes, without stirring.
11. Flip the fillets and immediately transfer the pan into the oven.
12. Bake for about 5-7 minutes or until desired doneness of salmon.
13. Divide the lentil mixture onto serving plates and top each with 1 salmon fillet.
14. Serve hot.

Salmon with Beans Salad

Prep Time 20 Min

Servings 4

Ingredients:
For Salmon
- 2 garlic cloves, minced
- 1 tablespoon fresh lemon zest, grated
- 2 tablespoons extra-virgin olive oil
- 2 tablespoons fresh lemon juice
- Salt and ground black pepper, as required
- 4 (6-ounce) boneless, skinless salmon fillets

For Dressing
- 5 tablespoons fresh orange juice
- 3 tablespoons extra-virgin olive oil
- 1 tablespoon red wine vinegar
- 1 tablespoon honey
- 1 tablespoon fresh orange zest, grated
- ¾ tablespoon Dijon mustard
- Salt and ground black pepper, as required

For Salad
- 3 cups cooked cannellini beans, rinsed and drained
- 6 cups fresh rocket
- 1 cup radishes, quartered
- 1 cup cherry tomatoes, halved
- ½ of red onion, finely sliced
- 2 tablespoons capers, rinsed

Directions:
1. Place all salmon Ingredients except for salmon fillets in a bowl and mix well.
2. Add the salmon fillets and coat with garlic mixture generously.
3. Preheat the grill to medium-high heat. Grease the grill grate.
5. Grill the salmon fillets onto the grill and cook for about 6-7 minutes per side.
6. Meanwhile, put all salad ingredients in a bowl and beat until well combined.
7. Mix all dressing ingredients and pour over salad.
8. Divide the beans salad onto serving plates and top each with 1 salmon fillet.
9. Serve immediately.

Tofu with Chickpeas & Kale

Prep Time 20 Min

Servings 4

Ingredients:
For Tofu
- 2 tablespoons extra-virgin olive oil
- 16 ounces tofu, drained, pressed, and cut into 1-inch cubes
- 1 tablespoon low-sodium soy sauce
- 1 teaspoon maple syrup
- 1 teaspoon red pepper flakes, crushed
- ¼ cup filtered water

For Chickpeas & Kale
- 2 tablespoons extra-virgin olive oil
- 3 cups cooked chickpeas, rinsed and drained
- ¼ teaspoon ground turmeric
- Salt and ground black pepper, as required
- 6 cups fresh baby kale
- 1 teaspoon sesame seeds

Directions:
1. Heat the olive oil over medium heat and cook the tofu cubes for about 8-10 minutes or until golden from all

sides.
2. Add the remaining ingredients and cook for about 2-3 minutes.
3. Meanwhile, in another sauté pan, heat the oil over medium heat and cook the chickpeas, turmeric, salt, and black pepper for about 2-3 minutes.
4. Remove the chickpeas from heat and transfer into a large bowl.
5. Add the tofu mixture and kale and stir to combine.
6. Garnish with sesame seeds and serve.

Beans & Veggie Salad

Prep Time 20 Min
Servings 4

Ingredients:
For Dressing
- 4 tablespoons extra-virgin olive oil
- 3 tablespoons fresh lime juice
- 1 tablespoon apple cider vinegar
- 2 tablespoons agave nectar
- Salt & Ground Black Pepper, As Required

For Salad
- 4 cups cooked red kidney beans, rinsed and drained
- 2 cups cherry tomatoes, halved
- 1 cup onion, sliced
- ¼ cup fresh parsley, minced
- 6 cups fresh baby kale

Directions:
1. Put all dressing ingredients in a small bowl and beat until well combined.
2. Next, put salad in a bowl, put all ingredients, and mix.
3. Add dressing and toss to coat well.
4. Serve immediately.

Buckwheat Noodles with Beef

Prep Time 20 Min
Servings 4

Ingredients:
For Steak
- 2 tablespoons extra-virgin olive oil
- 1 pound flank steak, sliced thinly
- Salt and ground black pepper, as required

For Salad
- 8 ounces buckwheat noodles
- 4 hard-boiled eggs, peeled and halved
- 1 cup radishes, cut into matchsticks
- 1 cup cucumber, cut into matchsticks
- 1 cup tomato, chopped
- ½ cup scallion greens, chopped
- 1 tablespoon sesame seeds

For Dressing
- ¼ cup fresh orange juice
- 3 tablespoons extra-virgin olive oil
- 2 tablespoons low-sodium soy sauce
- 2 tablespoons white vinegar
- 1 tablespoon fresh lime juice
- 1 tablespoon maple syrup
- 1 teaspoon fresh lime zest, grated
- 1 garlic clove, minced

Directions:
1. Heat oil in a large heavy-bottomed pan over medium-high heat and sear the beef slices with salt and black pepper for about 4-5 minutes or until cooked through.
2. Transfer the beef slices onto a plate and set aside.
3. Meanwhile, in a pan of lightly salted boiling water, cook the noodles for about 5 minutes.
4. Drain the noodles well and rinse under cold water.
5. Drain the noodles again.
6. For dressing: Put all ingredients in a bowl and beat until well combined.
7. Divide beef slices, noodles, veggies, and scallion into serving bowls and drizzle with dressing.
8. Garnish with sesame seeds and serve.

Buckwheat Noodles with Shrimp

Prep Time 20 Min
Servings 4

Ingredients:
- 10 ounces buckwheat noodles
- 5 tablespoons extra-virgin olive oil, divided
- 3 tablespoons low-sodium soy sauce
- 3 tablespoons balsamic vinegar
- 1 tablespoon Sriracha
- 1 tablespoon light brown sugar
- 1½ pounds raw shrimp, peeled and deveined
- Salt and ground black pepper, as required
- 1¾ cups zucchini, carrots, julienned
- 1¾ cups carrots, peeled and julienned

Directions:
1. Boil noodles in boiling water, cook the noodles for about 5 minutes. Drain and set aside.
2. Meanwhile in a bowl, add 3 tablespoons of oil, soy sauce, vinegar, Sriracha, and brown sugar and beat until well combined. Set aside.
3. Season the shrimp with salt and black pepper lightly.
4. Sautee shrimp in olive oil over medium-high heat and cook the shrimp for about 3-4 minutes, stirring occasionally.

5. Transfer the shrimp onto a plate.
6. In the same skillet, heat the remaining oil over medium-high heat and cook the zucchini and carrots for about 4-5 minutes, stirring occasionally.
7. Remove from heat, and toss with 3 tablespoons of the vinegar mixture.
8. For serving add noodles, shrimp, veggie mixture, and sauce and toss to coat well.
9. Serve immediately

Chicken Breast with Asparagus

Prep Time 10 Min
Cooking Time 20 min
Total Time 30 Min

Servings 4

Ingredients:
For Chicken
- ¼ cup extra-virgin olive oil
- ¼ cup fresh lemon juice
- 2 tablespoons maple syrup
- 1 garlic clove, minced
- Salt and ground black pepper, as required
- 5 (6-ounce) boneless, skinless chicken breasts

For Asparagus
- 1½ pounds fresh asparagus
- 2 tablespoons extra-virgin olive oil
- 1 tablespoon fresh lemon juice

DIRECTION
1. Add oil, lemon juice, Erythritol, garlic, salt, and black pepper in bowl and beat until well combined.
2. Marinate chicken in this mixture for 2 hours.
3. Preheat the grill to medium heat. Grease the grill grate.
4. Remove the chicken from the fridge and discard the marinade.
5. Place the chicken onto grill grate and grill, covered for about 5-8 minutes per side.
6. Place the asparagus in a steamer basket and steam, covered for about 5-7 minutes.
7. Drain the asparagus well and transfer into a bowl.
8. Add oil and lemon juice and toss to coat well.
9. Divide the chicken breasts and asparagus onto serving plates and serve.

Slow Cooker Salmon & walnut Soup

Prep Time 10 Min
Cooking Time 20 min
Total Time 30 Min

Servings: 4

Ingredients:
- 1 lb. salmon, cut into cubes
- 1 tbsp. Italian seasoning
- Salt and pepper, to taste
- 1/4 tsp. paprika powder
- 2 tbsps. olive oil
- 1 cup walnut milk
- parsley for topping

Directions:
1. Put all ingredients in a slow cooker and cook on low heat for 1 hour.
2. Once cooked remove from the cooker.
3. Drizzle parsley on top.
4. Serve and enjoy!

Salmon with Pesto & Beans

Prep Time 10 Min
Cooking Time 20 min
Total Time 30 Min

Servings: 2

Ingredients:
- 2 salmon fillet
- 1 tsp. garlic, minced
- 1 tbsp. Italian seasoning
- Salt and pepper, to taste
- 2 tbsps. olive oil
- green beans for serving
- lemon slice

Pesto sauce
- 1 cup basil leaves
- 1 garlic clove
- tbsp. lime juice
- pinch salt

Directions:
1. Toss salmon fillet with garlic, salt, pepper, and Italian seasoning.
2. Heat oil in a pan over medium heat.
3. Add salmon fillet and cook for 4-5 minutes.
4. Flip and cook for another 4-5 minutes until golden brown.
5. Sautee beans along with salmon fillet.
6. Once cooked remove from heat.
7. Meanwhile, blend pesto ingredients in a blender.
8. Drizzle pesto sauce over the salmon fillet.
9. Serve and enjoy!

Mushrooms & Kale Stew

Prep Time 10 min
Cooking time 30 min
Total time 40 min

Servings 4

Ingredients:
- 1/2 lb. mushroom, cut into halves

- 8 oz. kale, chopped
- salt & pepper to taste
- 1 tsp. cumin seeds
- 2 cups. vegetable broth
- 1 tbsp. olive oil
- 2-3 red chili, whole

Directions:
1. Heat the oil in a pan over medium heat
2. Once the oil is hot, add mushrooms and cook for 4-5 minutes until mushrooms are reduced.
3. Add kale and cook for 2-3 minutes
4. Season with salt, pepper, and other spices, and add broth and chilies.
5. Cover and cook over medium heat for about 15-20 minutes
6. Once cooked remove from heat.
7. Enjoy.

Grilled Crunchy Pepper

Prep Time 10 Min
Cooking Time 10 min
Total Time 20 Min

Servings 4

Ingredients:
- 1 green bell pepper, cut into thick slice
- 1 red bell pepper, cut into thick slice
- 1 yellow bell pepper, cut into thick slice
- 1 summer squash, sliced
- 1 carrot, peeled and roughly cut
- 1 tbsp. paprika
- Salt and pepper, to taste
- 2 tbsps. olive oil

Directions:
1. Season veggies with oil, salt, and pepper.
2. Preheat electric grill over medium heat.
3. Arrange veggies in greased grill grate.
4. Grill veggies for about 5-10 minutes until cooked through.
5. Serve and enjoy!

Stir Fried Shrimp & Kale

Prep Time 5 Min
Cooking Time 20 min
Total Time 25 Min

Servings: 4

Ingredients:
- 1 tsp garlic, minced
- 2 cup chopped kale
- 1 onion, chopped
- 1 lb. shrimp, trimmed
- ½ cup chopped tomatoes
- salt and pepper to taste
- 1 tbsp. olive oil
- 1 tbsps. lime juice

Directions:
1. Heat the oil in a pan over medium heat.
2. Once the oil is hot, add onion and garlic and cook for 2-3 minutes.
3. Add spinach in the same pan and cook for 5-6 minutes until kale is welted.
4. Add tomatoes and just cook for 2-3 minutes more.
5. Add shrimp and cook for 4-5 minutes until veggies are dried.
6. Once cooked remove from heat.
7. Drizzle lime juice on top.
8. Serve and enjoy!

Stir Fry Shrimp & Broccoli

Prep Time 5 Min
Cooking Time 15min
Total Time 20 Min

Servings 8

Ingredients:
- 1 broccoli head, cut into florets
- 1 cauliflower head, florets
- 2-3 carrots, sliced
- baby corn sliced
- lb. peeled and deveined shrimp
- 1 tbsp. extra virgin olive oil
- lemon juice
- 1 tsp. fresh chopped dill
- 1 tbsp. fresh chopped oregano
- ½ tsp smoked paprika
- ½ tsp sea salt
- ¼ tsp black pepper

Directions:
1. Heat your large frying pan over high heat, add oil.
2. Once the oil is hot, vegetables and fries for about 5-8 minutes.
3. Add dill, oregano, paprika, salt, and pepper, and mix well.
4. Add shrimp and cook covered for 5-8 minutes until all veggies are cooked through.
5. Once cooked remove from heat.
6. Drizzle lemon juice on top.
7. Serve and enjoy.

Chicken & Veggies Lunch Bowl

Prep Time 5 Min
Cooking Time 15 min
Total Time 20 Min

Servings 4

Ingredients:
- 1 chicken breast
- 1 tbsp. extra-virgin olive oil
- 1 red onion, finely sliced
- 4-5 fresh tomatoes, sliced
- kale leaves, chopped
- 1 lime juice
- salt & pepper to taste

Directions:
1. Coat chicken breast with oil, salt, and pepper all over. Grill chicken breast in a grill for about 5-10 minutes until cooked and brown.
2. Once cooked remove the breast from the grill.
3. Cut breast in bite-size pieces.
4. Assemble chopped kale leaves and tomato slices in a bowl.
5. Top with chicken breast.
6. Drizzle lime juice, salt, and pepper on top.
7. Serve and enjoy!

Lemon Fish Soup

Prep Time 10 Min
Cooking Time 20 min
Total Time 30 Min

Servings 4

Ingredients:
- 10 cups chicken broth
- 3 tbsps. olive oil
- 1 onion, chopped
- 1 large lemon, zested
- 2 salmon fillets in halves
- Salt and pepper
- ¼ cup green onion

Directions:
1. Heat the oil in a large pan over medium heat.
2. Add onion and cook for 2-3 minutes.
3. Add salmon cubes and cook for 4-5 minutes until cooked through.
4. Add chicken broth and season with salt, and pepper.
5. Bring broth to boil and simmer on low flame for about 20-25 minutes until chicken is cooked.
6. Sprinkle green onion and lime juice on top.
7. Serve immediately.
8. Enjoy!

Salmon & Potato Soup with Herbs

Prep Time 5 Min
Cooking time 40 Min
Total time 45 Min

Servings 6

Ingredients:
- 1 lb. salmon fillet cut into cubes
- 2-3 medium potatoes, cut into
- 2 tbsps. extra virgin olive oil
- 1 tbsp. onion powder.
- 1 tbsps. garlic powder
- 1/4 tsp. black pepper
- 1/2 tsp. salt
- warm water to cover
- 1 tbsp. lime juice

Directions:
1. Heat large heavy pot over medium heat, add oil.
2. Once the oil is hot, add salmon cubes and cook for about 4-5 minutes until cooked and no pinker.
3. Add tomatoes and cook for again 4-5 minutes.
4. Add onion, garlic powder, salt, and pepper in the same pot and mix well.
5. Add 6 cups of hot water to cover completely.
6. Cook covered for about 30 minutes to simmer on low heat.
7. Once cooked remove from heat.
8. Serve hot and enjoy!

Sweet Corn Soup with Herbs

Prep Time 5 Min

Cooking time 20 Min
Total time 25 Min

Servings: 4

Ingredients:
- 2 tbsp. olive oil
- 1 tsp. garlic, minced
- 1 can sweet corns, drained
- 6 cups chicken stock
- Salt to taste
- Pepper to taste
- 1 tbsp. lime juice
- Parsley

Directions:
1. Heat the oil in a large pot over medium heat.
2. Once the oil is hot, add garlic and sauté for about 1 minute.
3. Add sweet corns, broth and cook for about 3-4 minutes.
4. Season with salt and pepper and mix well.
5. Cover and cook on low heat for about 15 minutes.
6. Pour soup in a blender and blend for 5-10 seconds.
7. Pour soup into a serving bowl.
8. Top with some sweet corns and parsley and lime juice.
9. Enjoy!

Traditional Russian Cold Soup

Prep Time 10 Min
Cooking Time 20 Min
Total Time 30 Min

Servings: 4

Ingredients:
- 1 boil potato, chopped
- ¼ cup tomatoes, chopped
- 2 cups walnut cream
- 1 red onion, chopped
- 1 cucumber, chopped
- 1 oz. rosemary, chopped
- ⅛ tsp black pepper
- ¼ tsp salt
- 2 tbsps. olive oil

Directions:
1. Mix potato, tomato, onion, cucumber, and rosemary in a bowl.
2. Add walnut cream and mix well.
3. Season with salt and pepper, and mix well.
4. Drizzle olive oil on top.
5. Serve and enjoy!

Chicken Soup with Carrots

Prep Time 5 Min
Cooking Time 25 Min
Total Time 30 Min

Servings: 4

Ingredients:
- 1 chicken breast,
- 1 carrot, sliced
- 1 tbsp. olive oil
- 1 tsp garlic, minced
- 4 cups chicken broth
- Salt and pepper to taste
- ¼ cup parsley leaves

Directions:
1. Heat the oil in a 10-inch skillet, once the oil is hot, add chicken and garlic and cook for 3-4 minutes, until the chicken is no longer pink.
2. Season with salt, pepper, and mix well.
3. Add carrot and broth.
4. Cover and cook on low heat for 25-30 minutes until veggies are cooked.
5. Slightly shredded chicken with hand or spatula.
6. Sprinkle parsley leaves on top.
7. Serve and enjoy hot.

Chicken & Veggies Stew

Prep Time 10 Min
Cooking Time 20 Min
Total time 30 Min

Servings 4

Ingredients:
- 1 tbsp. olive oil
- 1/2 lb. chicken, boil and shredded
- 1 carrot, sliced
- ¼ cup green peas
- 4 cups chicken stock
- 1/2 tsp salt
- 1/4 tsp black pepper
- 1 tbsp. lime juice.
- 1/4 cup chopped parsley

Direction
1. Heat the olive oil in a non-stick soup pot over medium heat.
2. Once the oil is hot, add chicken, carrots, peas, and sauté for about 4-5 minutes.
3. Add the stock and season with salt, and pepper.
4. Cook covered for about 15-20 minutes on low heat until veggies are cooked through
5. Sprinkle lime juice on top.
6. Adjust seasoning according to taste and enjoy!

Lentils Soup with Kale

Prep Time 10 Min
Cooking time 20 Min
Total time 40 Min

Servings 4

Ingredients:
- 2 tbsps. olive oil
- 1 red onion, chopped
- 1/4 cup red lentils, soaked and drained
- 4 cups chicken broth
- salt & pepper to taste
- 2 cups kale

Topping
- 1 tomato, chopped
- 1 onion chopped
- Parsley
- 1 tbsps. lime juice

Directions:
1. Heat the oil in a saucepan over medium heat.
2. Once the oil is hot, add onion and cook for about 2-3 minutes.
3. Add lentils, broth, kale and cook covered for about 15-20 minutes.
4. Season with salt to taste mix well.
5. Add tomatoes, onion, parsley, and lime juice and mix well.
6. Serve and enjoy!

Cauliflower & Broccoli Soup

Prep Time 15 Min
Cooking Time 20 Min
Total Time 35 Min
Servings: 4

Ingredients:
- 1 medium broccoli florets
- 1 medium, cauliflower
- 1 tsp garlic, minced
- 1 tbsp. olive oil
- 4 cups chicken stock
- 1 tsp salt
- 1 tsp pepper
- 1 pinch curry powder
- 1 tbsp. parsley chopped
- 1 white onion, sliced

Directions:
1. Heat the oil in a pan over medium heat.
2. Once the oil is hot, cook broccoli and cauliflower with garlic for about 4-5 minutes.
3. Add broth and simmer on low to medium heat for 15-20 minutes.
4. Add in salt, pepper, curry powder, onion slice, and parsley.
5. Adjust seasoning to taste.
6. Serve hot and enjoy!

Shrimp Soup with Cream

Prep Time 05 Min
Cooking time 20 Min
Total time 25 Min
Servings: 4

Ingredients:
- 1 tbsp. olive oil
- 1 lb. shrimp,
- 2 cups kale chopped
- 1 tomato sliced
- 4 cups chicken stock
- 1 tsp. curry powder
- 1 cup walnut cream
- salt and pepper, to taste
- pinch of chili powder

Directions:
1. Heat the olive oil in a saucepan over medium heat.
2. Once the oil is hot, add shrimp and cook for another 2-3 minutes.
3. Season with salt, pepper, curry powder, chili powder, and add kale.
4. Add in cream, chicken stock, and mix well.
5. Cover and simmer for about 5-8 minutes on low heat.
6. Pour soup in a soup bowl with a tomato slice.
7. Drizzle lime juice on top.
8. Serve hot.

Kidney Beans & Tomato Soup

Prep Time 10 Min
Cooking time 30 Min
Total time 40 Min
Servings: 4

Ingredients:
- 2 tbsps. olive oil
- 1 can kidney beans, drained
- 1 cup tomato puree
- 1 cup tomato chopped
- 3 small onion rings
- 6 cups chicken stock
- salt and pepper to taste

Directions:
1. Place kidney beans, onion rings, stock, and tomato puree in a large stockpot over medium heat.
2. Bring to a simmer, cover, and cook for about 20 minutes, until the soup is thick.
3. Add salt, pepper and mix well.
4. Taste and add salt, if needed.
5. Add chopped tomatoes and serve.
6. Enjoy hot!

Walnut & Chicken Soup

Prep Time: 5 min
Cooking Time 25 min
Total Time 30 min
Servings 4

Ingredients
- 1 chicken breast, cut into cubes
- 1/2 lb. button mushrooms. sliced
- 1 cup walnut cream
- salt and pepper, to taste
- 6 cups. chicken stock
- 4-5 whole red pepper
- parsley

Directions:
1. Heat the oil in a pan, once the oil is hot, add chicken, cook for about 5-8 minutes until the chicken is no longer pink.
2. Add stock, red pepper, cream, and cook covered for about 8-10 minutes.
3. Season with salt and pepper and mix well.
4. Pour soup in bowls.
5. Serve and enjoy!

Shrimp & Zucchini Stew

Prep Time 5 Min
Cooking time 15 Min
Total time 20 Min
Servings: 4

Ingredients:
- 1 tbsp. olive oil
- 1 lb. shrimp, peeled
- 1 zucchini, roughly sliced
- 1 bunch kale, trimmed and chopped
- ¼ cup chopped onion
- ½ tsp. salt and pepper
- 4 cups chicken broth

Directions:
1. Heat the oil in a large pot over medium heat.
2. Once the oil is hot, add onion and sauté for about 2-3 minutes until onions are transparent.
3. Stir in the shrimp, zucchini, kale, chicken broth and season with salt and pepper.
4. Bring boil to a simmer for about 5-8 minutes until shrimp and veggies are cooked.
5. Sprinkle parsley leaves on top.
6. Enjoy!

Beans & Veggies Soup

Prep Time 5 Min
Cooking Time 25 Min
Total Time 30 Min
Servings: 4

Ingredients:
- 2 cups chopped broccoli
- 1 cup kale, chopped
- 1 cup kidney beans, drained
- 2 tbsps. onion powder
- 3 cups chicken stock
- 1 tbsp. olive oil
- 1/4 tsp. salt
- 1/8 tsp. pepper
- 1 tbsp. lime juice

Directions:
1. Heat oil in pan over medium heat.
2. Once oil is hot, add broccoli and carrot, cook for about 3-5 minutes, until veggies turn into brown.
3. Add stock, beans, kale, salt, pepper in pan and mix well.
4. Cover and cook on low heat for about 10-12 minutes until veggies are cooked through.
5. Drizzle lime juice on top.
6. Serve hot and enjoy!

French Lentils Soup

Prep Time 10 Min
Cooking Time: 20 Min
Total Time: 30 Min
Servings: 4

Ingredients
- 1 tbsp. olive oil
- 1 cup French lentils, soaked and drained
- Salt and pepper
- 1 tsp. garlic, minced
- 1 onion chopped
- 6 cups chicken broth
- salt and pepper to taste
- 1 tomato, chopped
- parsley chopped

Directions:
1. In a large saucepan over medium heat, heat the oil.
2. Sautee onion and garlic for about 3-4 minutes.
3. Add lentils, broth and bring to a boil, simmer for about 30-35 minutes until lentils are tendered.
4. Season with salt and pepper and mix well.
5. Top with tomato and parsley.
6. Drizzle lime juice on top.
7. Serve and enjoy!

Salmon & Beans Soup

Prep Time: 10 Min
Cooking Time: 25 Min
Total Time: 35 Min
Servings: 4

Ingredients
- 1 tbsp. olive oil
- 8 oz. green beans
- 1 carrot, chopped
- 1 salmon slice, cut into slice
- 1 garlic clove, minced
- 4 cups chicken stock
- 1/2 tsp salt
- 1/4 tsp black pepper

Directions:
1. Heat the oil in a nonstick soup pot, add salmon and cook with garlic for about 4-5 minutes.
2. Add the stock, beans, carrots, seasoning, and bring to boil, simmer for about 15 minutes.
3. Drizzle parsley lemon juice and mix well.
4. Serve and enjoy

Instant Pot Salmon Soup

Prep Time 5 Min
Cooking Time 20 Min

Total Time 25 Min

Servings 4

Ingredients:
- 1 salmon fillet cut into cubes
- 1/2 cup onion, chopped
- 1 bunch kale, chopped
- 1 tsp. garlic, minced
- 1 tsp. cumin seed powder
- ½ tsp. sea salt
- 2 tbsps. lemon juice
- 4 cups chicken broth

Topping
- 8 oz. walnut cream
- 1 oz. rosemary, chopped

Directions:
1. Put all ingredients into an Instant Pot.
2. Cover, close the lid, and cook on high pressure for about 18 minutes.
3. Allow pressure to release naturally, about 10 minutes, before removing the lid.
4. Add the rosemary and cream on top and stir well.
5. Serve immediately.

Instant Pot Beans Soup

Prep Time 5 Min
Cooking Time 20 Min
Total Time 25 Min

Servings 4

Ingredients:
- 1 cup kidney beans, boil
- 1 cup white beans, cooked
- 1 bunch kale, chopped
- 1 cup green onion, chopped
- 1 tsp. garlic, minced
- 1 tsp. cumin seed powder
- ½ tsp. sea salt
- 2 tbsps. olive oil
- 2 tbsps. lemon juice
- 4 cups water

Directions:
1. Put all ingredients with broth in an Instant Pot.
2. Cover, close the lid, and cook on high pressure for about 18 minutes.
3. Allow pressure to release naturally, about 10 minutes, before removing the lid.
4. Serve immediately.
5. Enjoy!

Detox Instant Veggies Stew

Prep Time 5 Min
Cooking time 5 Min
Total time 10 Min

Servings: 1

Ingredients:
- 1 carrot, sliced
- 8 oz. green beans
- 2 cups broccoli, florets
- 1 cup cauliflower, florets.
- 1 zucchini, sliced
- 1 cup green onion, chopped
- 1 tsp. garlic, minced
- 1 tbsp. curry powder
- 1 tsp. cumin seed powder
- ½ tsp. sea salt
- 2 tbsps. olive oil
- 2 tbsps. lemon juice
- 4 cups water

Directions:
1. Put all ingredients with broth in an Instant Pot.
2. Cover, close the lid, and cook on high pressure for about 18 minutes.
3. Allow pressure to release naturally, about 10 minutes, before removing the lid.
4. Serve immediately.
5. Enjoy!

Instant Chicken & Veggies Stew

Prep Time 10 Min
Cooking Time 20 Min
Total Time 30 Min

Servings: 6

Ingredients:
- 2 tbsps. garlic, minced
- 3 cups chicken broth
- 1 lb. mushrooms, halves
- 2 cups coconut cream
- 1 cup broccoli, florets
- ⅛ tsp white pepper
- ¼ tsp salt
- 2 tbsps. olive oil
- 1 green onion, sliced
- 4-5 cherry tomatoes

Directions:
1. Heat the oil in a pan over medium heat, add garlic and mushrooms and broccoli, cook until mushrooms and broccoli are brown and shrink.
2. Add chicken broth, cream salt, and pepper and cook for another 5-6 minutes over medium heat.
3. Once soup is cooked remove from heat.
4. Sprinkle green onion on top.

5. Enjoy!

Instant Pot Kale Stew

Prep Time 10 min
Cooking time 20 min
Total time 30 min

Servings 4

Ingredients:
- 1 onion, chopped
- 1 bunch kale, chopped \
- 2 cup cauliflower, roughly chopped
- 1 cup potato, chopped
- 1 cup green peas.
- 1 tsp garlic, minced
- 4 cups vegetable broth
- 2 tbsps. olive oil
- Salt, black pepper to taste
- 2 lime juice
- 1/2 cup parsley, chopped

Directions:
1. Put all ingredients with broth in an Instant Pot.
2. Cover, close the lid, and cook on high pressure for about 18 minutes.
3. Allow pressure to release naturally, about 10 minutes, before removing the lid.
4. Add chopped parsley on top and stir well.
5. Serve immediately.

Dessert & Snacks Recipes

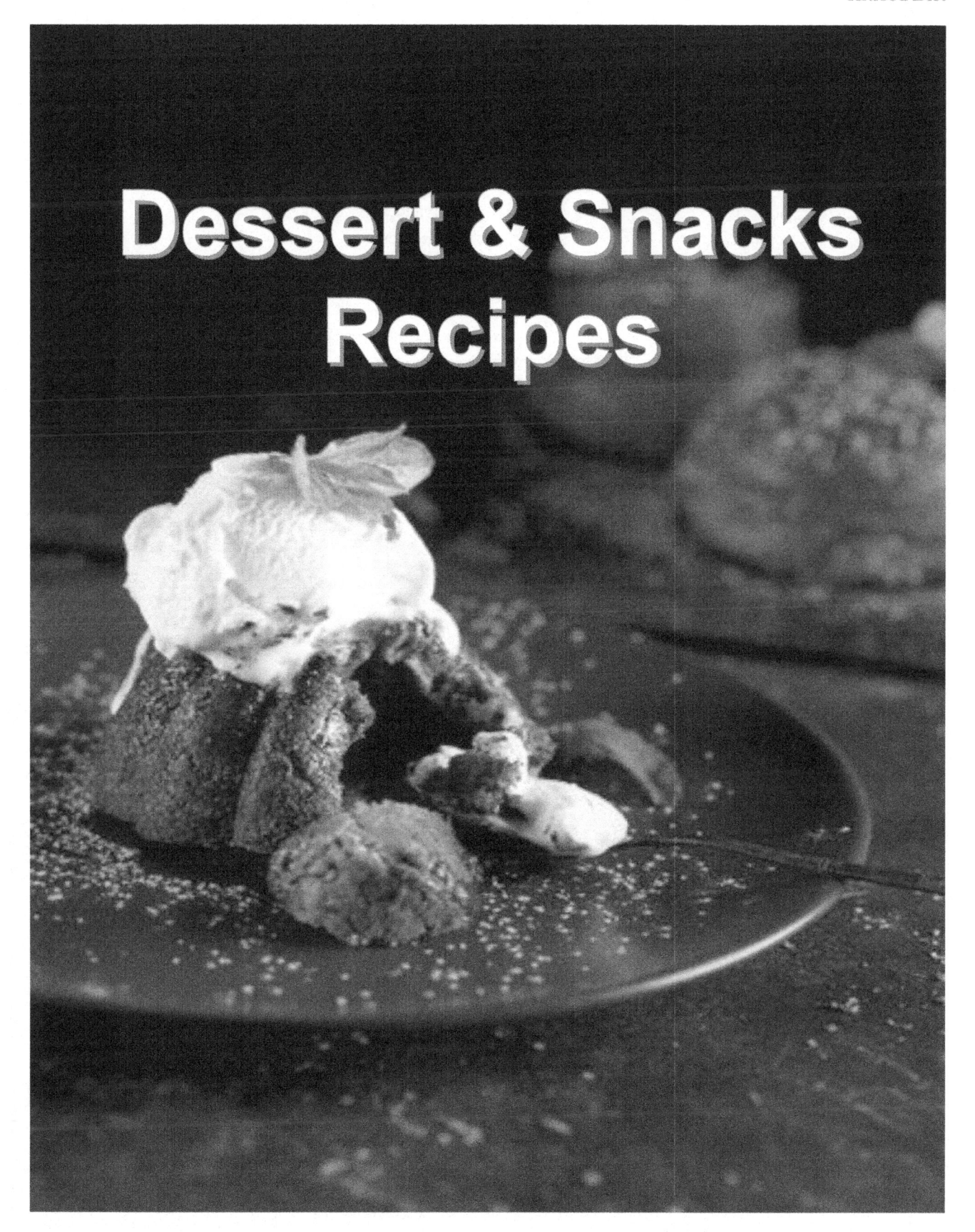

Apple & Walnuts Cake

Prep Time 50 Min

Servings 16

Ingredients:
- 8 cups sliced peeled tart apples
- 1 cup dates syrup
- 2 cups walnuts milk
- 2 teaspoons ground cinnamon
- 1 cup walnut butter, softened
- 2 cups buckwheat flour
- 1 cup finely chopped walnuts, divided

Directions:
1. Place apples in a greased 13x9-in baking dish.
2. Sprinkle with cinnamon.
3. Mix flour, milk, syrup, and walnuts in a bowl.
4. Pour mixture over apples. Sprinkle with remaining walnuts.
5. Bake at 350° for 45-55 minutes.
6. Serve and enjoy!

Nutritional information:
Calories Per Servings, 293 kcal, 16.37 g Fat, 36.89 g Total Carbs, 3.89 g Protein, 3.3 g Fiber

Baked Walnut Brownies

Prep Time 30 Min

Servings 16

Ingredients:
- 4 tablespoons walnuts butter
- 3/4 cup buckwheat flour
- 1/2 teaspoon salt
- 3/4 teaspoon baking powder
- 1/8 teaspoon baking soda
- 1 cup dates chopped
- ¼ cup dates syrup
- 1 cup walnuts (chopped)

Directions:
1. Preheat oven to 350 F.
2. Grease brownies pan with cooking spray.
3. In a medium bowl, mix the dry ingredients until well incorporated.
4. Blend the dates, melted butter, dates, and walnuts in a blender.
5. Stir in flour mixture until well blended.
6. Pour the thick batter into the prepared baking pan and spread it evenly with a spatula.
7. Bake in the preheated oven for about 20 to 24 minutes, or until browned and the top has formed a crust.
8. Slice it.
9. Serve cold and enjoy!

Nutritional information:
Calories Per Servings, 170 kcal, 6.57 g Fat, 27.85 g Total Carbs, 2.12 g Protein, 2.1 g Fiber

Coco & Walnuts Smoothie

Prep Time 10 Min

Servings 1

Ingredients:
- 1 cup soy milk
- 1 tsp dates syrup
- 1/2 oz. walnuts
- 1 tbsp. cocoa powder
- 1/2 cup ice cubes

Directions:
1. Put all ingredients in a high-speed blender.
2. Blend until all ingredients are incorporated.
3. Serve and enjoy!

Nutritional information:
Calories Per Servings, 262 kcal, 17.25 g Fat, 16.09 g Total Carbs, 9.85 g Protein, 1 g Fiber

Walnut Cream Cake

Prep Time 40 Min

Servings 10

Ingredients:
- 4 oz. buckwheat flour
- 1 teaspoon baking powder
- 4 oz. walnut cream
- ¼ cup dates syrup
- 1 cup soy milk
- 2 oz. walnut, chopped

Directions:
1. Grease cake pan with cooking oil or olive oil
2. Mix the flour and baking powder, set aside.
3. Add dates syrup and the rest of the ingredients in the flour and mix well.
4. Pour the batter into the greased pan, shake gently to level off the batter.
5. Bake at a pre-heated oven at 180C (350F) for about 30-35 minutes or until cooked.
6. Serve and enjoy!

Nutritional information:
Calories Per Servings, 195 kcal, 14.06 g Fat, 16.51 g Total Carbs, 3.16 g Protein, 1.5 g Fiber

Walnuts Bits

Prep Time 40 Min

Servings 20

Ingredients:
- 1/2 cup walnut butter softened
- 8 oz. walnut cream
- 1/2 cup dates, finely chopped
- 1 cup walnuts, chopped
- 1/2 cup dates, chopped
- 2 tbsps. sesame seeds

Directions:
1. In a large bowl, mix all ingredients except chopped dates and sesame seeds.
2. Gently fold in chopped dates.
3. Use a cookie scoop to make 20 even bites and place onto prepared cookie sheet.
4. Roll on sesame seeds.
5. Place in fridge for 30 minutes - 1 hour, or until firm.
6. Serve and enjoy!

Nutritional information:
Calories Per Servings, 185 kcal, 17.04 g Fat, 7.47 g Total Carbs, 2.92 g Protein, 1.9 g Fiber

Walnuts Bites Muffins

Prep Time 40 Min

Servings 12

Ingredients:
- 1/2 cup dates sugar
- 2 cups buckwheat flour
- 2 teaspoons baking powder
- 1/2 teaspoon salt
- 2/3 cup soy milk
- 1/2 cup walnut butter, melted, cooled
- 1 cup dark chocolate, melted
- 1/2 cup California walnuts, chopped

Directions:
1. Preheat oven to 400°F. Grease or line 12 large muffin cups.
2. In a large bowl, mix sugars, buckwheat flour, baking powder, and salt. In a medium bowl, combine milk, butter, chocolate and blend well.
3. Mix dry ingredients with wet ingredients.
4. Pour batter into greased muffin cups.
5. Bake for 15 to 20 minutes or until cooked.
6. Serve hot and enjoy!

Nutritional information:
Calories Per Servings, 271 kcal, 18.37 g Fat, 23.85 g Total Carbs, 5.51 g Protein, 4.7 g Fiber

Buckwheat Cinnamon Buns

Prep Time 30 Min

Servings 8

Ingredients:
- 14-16 oz. buckwheat dough
- 1 cup dates syrup
- 2 tbsps. cinnamon powder,
- 2 tbsps. walnut butter, melted

Directions:
1. Preheat oven to 400 degrees F.
2. Roll dough into a rectangle about 10 X 14 inches.
3. Mix syrup and cinnamon powder in a mixing bowl.
4. Spread this mixture over rolled dough.
5. Roll dough in a circle.
6. Slice dough with knife or pizza cutter into 1-inch pieces. Place rolls on prepared sheets.
7. Quickly brush butter over rolls.
8. Bake rolls for about 15 minutes or until lightly brown and rolls are cooked through.

Nutritional information:
Calories Per Servings, 170 kcal, 0.41 g Fat, 43.33 g Total Carbs, 1.8 g Protein, 1.4 g Fiber

Dates Brownies Bars

Prep Time 40 Min

Servings 12

Ingredients:
- 2 cup dates, chopped
- ¼ cup dates syrup
- 1 tsp. baking powder
- 1 tsp. sea salt
- ½ cup walnut butter, melted
- ½ cup walnut milk
- 1/2 cup cocoa powder

Directions:
1. Preheat oven to 350°.
2. In a large bowl mix all ingredients and blend in blender.
3. Pour brownies mixture in lined brownies mold.
4. Bake in preheated oven for about 20 minutes until cooked.
5. Slice it and drizzle chocolate syrup on top.
6. Serve and enjoy!

Nutritional information:
Calories Per serving 156 Cal, Fats 8.97 g, Protein 3.66 g, Total Carbs 19 g, Fiber 3.3 g

Chocolate Pudding With Berries

Prep Time 5 min

Servings 4

Ingredients:
- 2 cups walnut milk
- 2 tbsps. chia seeds
- 2 tbsps. cocoa powder

- 1 tsp dates syrup
- fresh berries, coconut flake for topping

Directions:
1. Mix milk with dates syrup, chia seeds, and cocoa powder in a bowl and mix well.
2. Pour in serving jar and let it stand overnight in the fridge.
3. In the morning, top pudding with berries.
4. Serve and enjoy!

Nutritional information:
Calories Per serving 136 Cal, Fats 13.05 g, Protein 3.05 g, Total Carbs 4.11 g, Fiber 1.3 g

Dark Chocolate Cookies

Prep Time 30 min

Servings 12

Ingredients:
- 1/4 cup walnut butter
- 2 tbsps. walnut cream
- 2 cup buckwheat flour
- 1 pinch. sea salt
- 1 tbsps. date syrup
- 3/4 cup cocoa powder

Directions:
1. Preheat the oven to 350°.
2. Mix all ingredients in a bowl and knead the dough for 5 minutes.
3. Divide the dough into 15 equal balls.
4. Shape the ball and flatten the balls on a greased baking tray.
5. Bake chocolate cookies for about 15-20 minutes in the preheated oven until cooked and crispy.
6. Serve and enjoy!

Nutritional information:
Calories Per serving 194 Cal, Fats 11.26 g, Protein 3.68 g, Total Carbs 21.08 g, Fiber 3.6 g

Homemade Walnut Milk

Prep Time 5 Min

Servings 4

Ingredients:
- 1 cup walnuts
- 2 cups water
- 1/4 tsp cinnamon

Directions:
1. Soak walnuts in freshwater for 8 hours or overnight or for at least 8 hours.
2. Drain the walnuts and place walnuts with fresh water and cinnamon in an electric blender.
3. Blend walnuts for about 1-2 minutes.
4. Strain milk and store it in the fridge.
5. Serve and enjoy!

Nutritional information:
Calories Per Servings, 131 kcal, 13.04 g Fat, 3.05 g Protein, 2.88 g Total Carbs, 1.4 g Fiber

Apple & Spinach Smoothie

Prep Time 10 Min

Servings 1

Ingredients:
- 1 cup walnuts milk
- 1 tsp dates syrup
- 1 apple, chopped
- 1 cup spinach
- 1 pinch cinnamon

Directions:
1. Put all ingredients in a high-speed blender.
2. Blend until all ingredients are incorporated.
3. Serve and enjoy!

Nutritional information:
Calories Per Servings, 169 kcal, 13.23 g Fat, 3.43 g Protein, 12.55 g Total Carbs, 2.5 g Fiber

Homemade Walnut Cream

Prep Time 10 Min

Servings 4

Ingredients:
- 2 cups California walnuts
- 1 cup water

Directions:
1. Pour walnuts and water in a high-power blender or food processor until the mixture is very smooth and fluffy.
2. Store in an airtight jar and use in desserts.
3. Enjoy!

Nutritional information:
Calories Per Servings, 262 kcal, 26.08 g Fat, 6.08 g Protein, 5.48 g Total Carbs, 2.7 g Fiber

Homemade Walnut Butter

Prep Time 30 Min

Servings 4

Ingredients:
- 1-1/2 cups walnuts

Directions:
1. Roast the walnuts in preheated oven or pan for about 12 minutes until golden brown.

2. Pour the walnut in a blender and processor for 1-2 minutes.
3. Scrape and blend for another 1-3 minutes.
4. Store butter in an airtight container and use it in desserts.

Nutritional information:
Calories Per Servings, 196 kcal, 19.56 g Fat, 4.57 g Protein, 4.11 g Total Carbs, 2 g Fiber

Cinnamon Chocolate Bites

Prep Time 15 min

Servings 8

Ingredients:
- ½ cup walnuts
- ¼ cup dark chocolate
- cup Medjool dates, pitted
- 1 tbsp. cocoa powder
- 1 tbsp. cinnamon powder
- 1 tbsp. extra virgin olive oil
- water

Directions:
1. Place all the ingredients in a food processor and mix well.
2. Add water if required. The mixture should not be sticky.
3. Form walnut-sized balls with your hands and roll over cocoa powder.
4. Roll balls on cinnamon powder.
5. Freeze balls in the freezer.
6. Once set serve and enjoy!

Nutritional information:
Calories Per Servings, 95 kcal, 7.16 g Fat, 1.61 g Protein, 7.37 g Total Carbs, 1.8 g Fiber

Walnut Ice-cream

Prep Time 10 min

Servings 2

Ingredients:
- 1 cup walnut cream
- 2 oz. walnuts
- ¼ cup dates syrup

Directions:
1. Freeze walnut cream in the freezer.
2. Scoop walnut cream in bowl top with walnuts and dates syrup.
3. Serve immediately.
4. Enjoy!

Nutritional information:
Calories per serving 173 Cal, Fats 13.29 g, Protein 3.59 g, Total Carbs 13.46 g, Fiber 3.1 g

Walnut Cream Smoothie

Prep Time 10 min

Servings 2

Ingredients:
- cup raspberries
- 1 cup walnut cream
- 1 cup ice cubes
- ¼ cup fresh raspberries for topping

Directions:
1. Pour raspberries, ice-cream, and cream in an electric high-speed blender and blend.
2. Pour creamy smoothie in serving jar.
3. Top with raspberries.
4. Serve cold and enjoy!

Nutritional information:
Calories per serving 178 Cal, Fats 2.16 g, Protein 3.78 g, Total Carbs 38.77 g, Fiber 1.8 g

Blueberries Smoothie

Prep Time 10 min

Servings 1

Ingredients:
- 1/2 cup frozen blueberries
- ½ cup soy milk
- 1 cup ice cubes

Directions:
1. Mix all the ingredients into a blender, blend until thick and creamy
2. Pour smoothie in serving glass and top with fresh blueberries.
3. Enjoy!

Nutritional information:
Calories per serving 113 Cal, Fats 3.1 g, Protein 2.64 g, Total Carbs 20.04 g, Fiber 3.2 g

Sirtfood Dates Bites

Prep Time 20 Min

Servings 20

Ingredients:
- 16 oz. chocolate
- 1 cup walnut cream
- 1 cup chopped dates

Directions:
1. Mix all ingredients in a bowl.
2. Let the mixture sit for 15 minutes.
3. Freeze the mixture for 2 hours until firm.
4. Scoop or spoon the mixture into small balls and roll-on cocoa powder.

5. Refrigerate the rolled truffles for 2 hours.
6. Serve and enjoy!

Nutritional information:
Calories per serving 359 Cal, Fats 26.04 g, Protein 14.5 g, Total Carbs 22.31 g, Fiber 10.1 g

Tofu & Blueberries Pie

Prep Time 60 Min

Servings 10

Ingredients:
- 1 cup buckwheat flour
- 1 oz walnut butter
- 1 cup apple puree
- 1/2 cup walnut cream
- 1 cup tofu, crumbled
- 1/4 cup dates syrup
- 1/4 tsp Sea salt
- 1 tsp Vanilla extract
- 1 cup blueberry puree

Directions:
1. Mix the flour and butter in a bowl.
2. Press the crust into the bottom of the greased pan. Keep the pan in the fridge.
3. Meanwhile, mix cream, tofu, dates syrup salt, and vanilla until smooth and fluffy.
4. Pour the half-filling into the crust, then pour blueberry puree and then the remaining mixture.
5. Gently tap on the counter to release air bubbles.
6. Bake in preheated oven for 40-50 minutes, until the pie is almost set.
7. Cool completely on the counter, then refrigerate at least an hour before slicing. Pie can be refrigerated overnight.

Nutritional information:
Calories per serving 114 kcal, Fats 6.03 g, Protein 3.8 g, Total Carbs 14.44 g, Fiber 3 g

Matcha Green Tea Bar

Prep Time 60 Min

Servings 10

Ingredients:
- ½ cup walnut butter
- 1 cup walnut milk
- 1 cup buckwheat flour
- 4 tbsps. matcha powder
- ⅛ tsp salt

Directions:

1. Line an 8x8" brownie pan with parchment paper. Set aside.
2. Put all of the ingredients in an electric stand mixer and mix well.
3. Scoop the mixture into the brownie pan and flatten it out.
4. Tightly cover the pan with plastic wrap and refrigerate overnight.
5. Lift the mixture out of the pan.
6. Slice into 12 bars.
7. Enjoy!

Nutritional information:
Calories per serving 182 kcal, Fats 6.84 g, Protein 16.9 g, Total Carbs 14.52 g, Fiber 1.5 g

Easy Walnut Milk

Prep Time 5 Min

Servings 4

Ingredients:
- 1 cup walnuts
- 3 cups filtered water
- 1/4 tsp cinnamon

Directions:
1. Soak walnuts in water for 8 hours or overnight.
2. night for at least 8 hours.
3. In the morning, strain the walnuts and place them with filtered water and cinnamon in a blender.
4. Blend for 1-2 minutes.
5. Strain milk and store in fridge for 3-4 days.
6. Serve and enjoy!

Nutritional information:
Calories Per Servings, 131 kcal, 13.04 g Fat, 3.05 g Protein, 2.88 g Total Carbs, 1.4 g Fiber

Healthy Berries Smoothie Bowl

Prep Time 10 min

Servings 2

Ingredients:
- 1 cup walnut cream
- 1 cup raspberries

Topping
- 2 oz. strawberries, sliced
- 2 oz. raspberries
- 1 oz. pumpkin seeds

Directions:
1. Add cream and raspberries in an electric blender.
2. Blend well until creamy and smooth.
3. Top with raspberries, strawberries, and pumpkin seeds.
4. Serve and enjoy!

Kale & Walnut Dip

Prep Time 20 min

Servings 6

Ingredients:
- 1 cup kale
- 1 cup mint leaves
- 1 garlic clove
- ¼ cup walnuts
- 1 lime juice
- salt and pepper

Directions:
1. Blend all ingredients in a high-speed blender for 1 minute.
2. Serve and enjoy!

Chocolate & Avocado Spread

Prep Time 20 min

Servings 6

Ingredients:
- 2 cups walnut cream
- 2 tbsps. coconut oil
- ¼ cup cocoa powder
- 1 avocado

Directions:
1. Blend all ingredients in a high-speed blender for 1 minute.
2. Serve and enjoy!

Chicken Snacks

Prep Time 15 Min
Cooking Time 10 min
Total Time 25 Min

Servings: 4

Ingredients:
- 2 chicken breast, ground
- 1/2 cup buckwheat flour
- 2 tbsps. onion powder
- 2 tbsps. garlic powder
- 1 tsp. dried oregano
- 1 tsp. paprika powder
- 1 tsp. salt
- 1/2 tsp. black pepper
- 2 tbsps. olive oil

Directions:
1. Mix flour, onion, garlic powder, oregano, paprika powder, salt, black pepper, and chicken in a bowl and set aside.
2. Make oval kebab by this mixture,
3. Heat the oil in a 10-inch skillet, add oil.
4. Once the oil is hot, place the chicken kebab in skillet and cook for 6-8 minutes.
5. Serve with BBQ sauce and enjoy.

Garlic & Cucumber Dip

Prep Time: 10 min

Servings: 4

Ingredients:
- 1 cucumber, chopped
- 1 tsp. garlic, minced
- 1 tbsp. chopped shallot
- 2 tsps. olive oil
- 1/2 tsp. Italian seasoning
- 1/8 tsp. salt
- 1 cup mint leaves
- 1 cup walnut cream

Directions:
1. Put all ingredients in a food processor except cream and blend until mixed.
2. Mix this paste with cream in a mixing bowl.
3. Adjust salt according to taste.
4. Serve and enjoy!

Chocolate Smoothie Jar

Prep Time 10 min

Servings 2

Ingredients:
- 1 cup walnut milk
- ¼ cup cocoa powder
- 2 tbsps. chia seeds
- **TOPPING**
- Strawberries

Directions:
1. Mix milk, chia seeds, and cocoa powder in a bowl and leave overnight in the fridge.
2. In the morning top smoothie with strawberries slice.
3. Serve and enjoy!

Beet Root & Kale Hummus

Prep Time: 10 min

Servings: 4

Ingredients:
- 1/4 cup walnut butter
- 1/4 cup lemon juice
- 1 tbsp. olive oil
- 1 cup kale chopped
- 1 cup beetroot, chopped
- 1/4 tsp. sea salt

- 1/4 tsp. cayenne pepper
- 1/4 tsp. ground turmeric
- 1 tbsp. parsley, chopped

Directions:
1. Put all ingredients in a food processor and blend until mixed. Once mixed, pour in a bowl.
2. Adjust salt according to taste.
3. Drizzle olive oil, chickpeas and sesame seeds on top
4. Serve and enjoy!

Walnut Dip

Prep Time: 5 min

Servings: 4

Ingredients:
- 1/4 cup walnuts, sacked whole night
- 4 cloves garlic, chopped
- 2 tbsps. fresh lemon juice
- 1 tbsp. olive oil
- ¾ cup water
- 2 tbsps. fresh parsley leaves salt and pepper to taste

Directions:
1. Put all ingredients in a blender and blend.
2. Process until a paste is smooth and fluffy.
3. Season with salt and pepper and mix well.
4. Serve with chicken nuggets.

Turmeric & Olives Hummus

Prep Time 10 Min

Servings: 8

Ingredients:
- 1/4 cup tahini
- 1/4 cup lemon juice
- 1 tbsp. olive oil
- 1/2 cup capers
- 1 tbsp. nutritional yeast
- 1/4 tsp. sea salt
- 1/4 tsp. cayenne pepper
- 1/4 tsp. ground turmeric
- 1 tbsp. parsley, chopped

Directions:
1. Put all ingredients in a high-speed food processor and mix thoroughly.
2. If the dressing seems too thick, add a little more water.
3. Top with cayenne and chopped parsley.
4. Serve and enjoy!

Chocolate Whipped Cream

Prep Time 10 Min

Servings: 10

Ingredients:
- 3 cups coconut cream cold
- 1/2 cup cocoa powder
- 1/2 cup coconut sugar

Directions:
1. Beat cream with blender, add sugar and cocoa powder, and beat again for 5-10 minutes.
2. Serve on ice cream or toast.

Creamy Avocado Sauce

Prep Time 10 Min

Servings: 10

Ingredients:
- 3 cups walnut cream cold
- 1 lime juice
- 1 tsp. garlic, mashed
- 2 avocados mashed

Directions:
1. Beat cream with blender and beat for 5-10 minutes.
2. Add the rest of the ingredients and beat again.
3. Serve on ice cream or toast.

Healthy Matcha Tea Smoothie

Prep Time 10 min

Servings 2

Ingredients:
- 1/2 cup walnut cream
- 1 cup avocado chopped
- 1 cup mint leaves
- 1 tbsp. matcha green tea powder

Topping
- 1 kiwi fruit, sliced
- 2 oz. blueberries
- 2 oz. raspberries
- 1 oz. chopped nuts
- 1 oz. pumpkin seeds

Directions:
1. Add cream, avocado, mint, and green tea powder in an electric blender.
2. Blend well until creamy and smooth.
3. Top with kiwi slice, blueberries, raspberries, nuts, and pumpkin seeds.
4. Serve and enjoy!

Spicy Shrimp Wrap

Prep Time: 5 min
Cooking Time: 20 min
Total Time: 25 min

Servings: 4

Ingredients:
- 4 buckwheat tortillas
- 1 lb. shrimp, peeled
- 5-8 cherry tomatoes, cut into two
- 1/2 tsp Italian seasoning
- 1 avocado, chopped
- ½ cup green peas
- 1 tbsp. olive oil
- arugula leaves
- 1 lemon, sliced

Directions:

1. Heat the oil in a pan over medium heat.
2. Once the oil is hot, add shrimp and cook for 4-5 minutes until cooked.
3. Season with Italian seasoning and mix well.
4. Once cooked remove from heat.
5. Toss the tortilla on a griddle for 2-3 minutes.
6. Lay the tortilla on a plate.
7. Spread arugula leaves on each tortilla.
8. Divide shrimp, avocado, tomatoes, and peas on each tortilla.
9. Drizzle lime juice, paprika on each tortilla and serve!

28 days Sirtfood Diet Plan & Guide Book

COPYRIGHT

All rights reserved. No part of this publication may be distributed, transmitted, or reproduced by any means or in any form, including photocopying, recording, or other electronic or mechanical methods, without the permission of the publisher, except in the case of brief quotations embodied in critical reviews and specific other noncommercial uses acceptable by copyright law.

Table of Contents

Introduction 111
    What Is Sirtfood Diet Plan? 111
    What Are Sirtfoods? 111
    Benefits Of Sirtfood Diet 111
        Weight-Loss *111*
        Anti-Aging: *112*
        Detoxification *112*
        Controls Blood Sugar Levels: *112*
        Improved Metabolism *112*
    How Does Sirtfood Diet Work? 113
    Phase I Of Sirtfood Diet 113
    Phase Ii Of Sirtfood Diet 113
    Sirtfood Green Juice 113
        Extra-Virgin Olive Oil *114*
        Soy *114*
        Rocket Or Arugula *114*
        Strawberries *114*
        Kale *115*
        Blueberries *115*
        Red Wine *115*
        Green Tea *115*
        Turmeric *116*
        Coffee *116*
        Onions *116*
        Walnuts *116*
        Buckwheat *117*
        Parsley *117*
        Chili *117*
        Medjool Dates *117*
        Celery *118*
        Lovage *118*
        Dark Chocolate *118*
    Foods To Avoid Having On The Sirtfood Diet 119
    Sirtfood Diet For Vegans 119
    Sirtfood Diet And Diabetics 119
    Sirtfood Diet And Pcos 119
    Sirtfood Diet & Alcohol 119
    Sirtfood Diet & Oats 119

Sirtfood Diet 120

28- Days Meal Plan 120
    Week-1 Sirtfood Meal Plan 121
    Week-2 Sirtfood Meal Plan 121
    Week-3 Sirtfood Meal Plan 122
    Week-4 Sirtfood Meal Plan 122

INTRODUCTION

WHAT IS SIRTFOOD DIET PLAN?

The sirtfood diet is going to be popular because it is effective for those who just couldn't achieve weight-loss through dieting or strenuous exercises. This diet is perfect for those who are battling with overweight due to genetic problems or low metabolic rates, and thus desire weight loss formula. The diet, therefore, not only recommends a calorie restriction but also provides a gradual stepwise process that helps activate the 'skinny genes. The combination of sirtfood and its two phases of diet makes a complete package that is known as a diet plan.

The sirtfood diet only restricts the calorie intake for the first phase in the diet plan; it never excludes any of the major ingredients from your diet. This diet promotes and suggests more intake of those food items that can help the activation of sirtuins. This diet suggests consumption of more green leafy vegetables, healthy fruits, grains, etc. This diet offers a lot of healthy food items that are easily available and affordable.

WHAT ARE SIRTFOODS?

The sirtfoods activate Sirtuins like polyphenols in a sufficient amount. There are many commonly used food items in our daily routine that can provide enough polyphenols to stimulate the sirtuins in your body. Such food items are berries, green tea, turmeric, dark chocolate, parsley, kale, capers, red wine, arugula, chilies, walnuts, olive oil, onions, etc. These ingredients do not share a single group of food, they vary in their origin and nutritional values, but the only thing that is common to them is the presence of polyphenol compounds like kaempferol, resveratrol, quercetin, etc. It's not that the Sirtfood dieter can only rely on these sirtfoods while on this diet, they can consume other food items as well as long as that don't disturb the calorie restriction prescribed by the diet and high sirtfood intake is also maintained.

BENEFITS OF SIRTFOOD DIET

The sirtfood diet offers several health benefits besides weight-loss. And these benefits are linked with the activation of sirtuins in the body. Many health experts state that high amounts of Sirtuins slow down aging.

The following health benefits can be achieved while considering the role of Sirtuin in the body

Weight-loss

During the first phase of this diet plan, a person can easily lose up to 7 pounds of his weight through calorie restriction. Up to 8-9 pounds weight can be loosed by the end of the three weeks of this diet. But the decrease in weight loss varies from person to person. Some people experience weight loss during the early days of the diet, whereas some can achieve their target by the end of this diet plan.

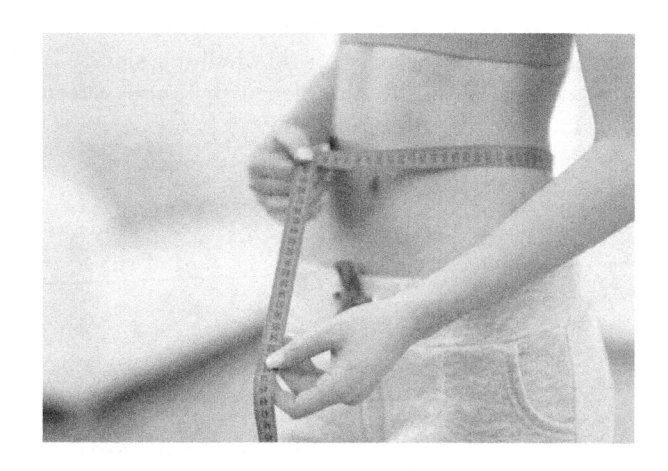

Anti-Aging:

Aging is linked to the life cycle of our cells. The cells of our body lose their ability to repair, heal, or reproduce quickly after a certain age, and that results in a condition known as aging. There are certain ways in which diet, environmental conditions, and lifestyle influence the process of aging; an unhealthy lifestyle speeds up this process. However, higher Sirtuin activity in the cells can slow down aging, and it helps produce new healthy cells in the body. Thus, a sirtfood diet and Sirtuin activators can help you stay young and healthy for long.

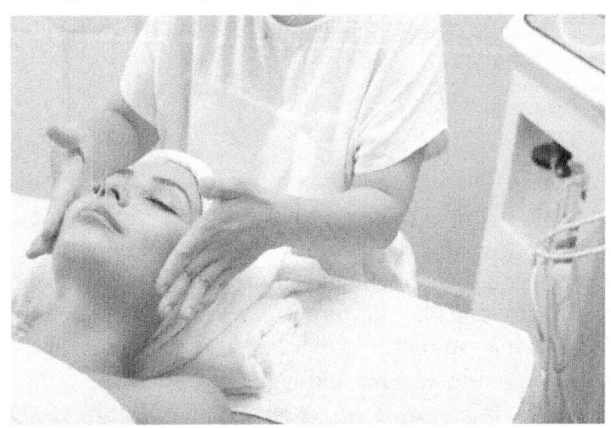

Detoxification

The sirtfood diet offers several ingredients that are full of antioxidants like green tea, red wine, onions, parsley, spinach, and several others are found in sirtfood. Antioxidants basically remove all the toxic material or oxidants that can damage the cell or slows down its metabolism. Antioxidants boost cellular activity and help the cells get rid of all the metabolic wastes. Therefore, the Sirt diet, with healthy green juices, offers regular detoxification.

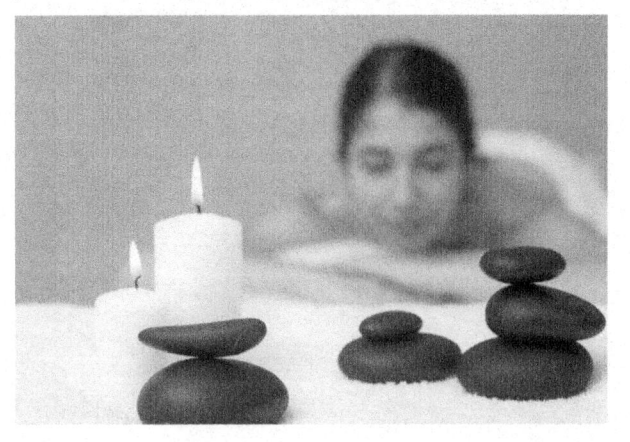

Controls Blood Sugar levels:

Sirtfood diet recommends calorie restriction, forces you to skip meals that are full of sugars and excessive carbohydrates; you can only eat healthy food with clean energy. Living on such food items can maintain your blood sugar levels and prevents insulin resistance in the body.

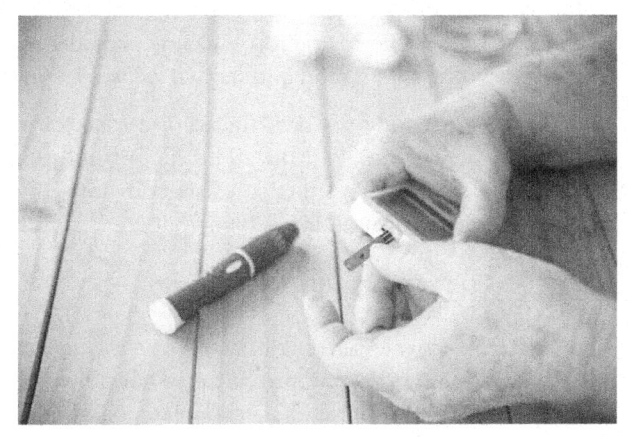

Improved Metabolism

Sirtuins directly affect the metabolic rates of the body. The sirtfood diet boosts the metabolic rates of the body by stimulating the sirtuins. That's why when a person lives on the sirtfood diet, more calories and fats are burnt with lesser physical activity.

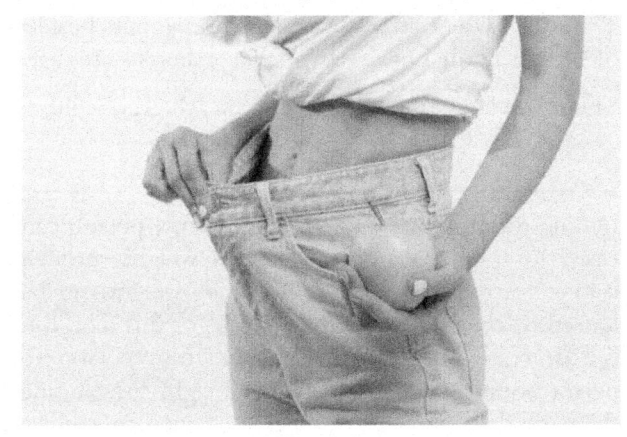

HOW DOES SIRTFOOD DIET WORK?

The sirtfood diet plan is mainly divided into two different phases of diet plan. The basic purpose is to slowly introduce the changes that can help stimulate the Sirtuin activities and aid weight loss. The first phase is thought to be more difficult than the second phase because of its calorie restriction. But you can reduce more weight in the first phase.

The main goal of calorie restriction is to activate the sirtuins, and it occurs when we reduce calories first and then provide the Sirtuin activators to the body. These two phases work together, hand in hand, in order to achieve all of its benefits. The three-week sirtfood diet plan is divided into two phases according to the following dietary guidelines.

PHASE I of Sirtfood Diet

Phase I of the sirtfood diet lasts for the first seven days. This is the stage in which dieters will have to embark on calorie restriction and consume green juice in large quantities. For the first three days, the dieter needs to live on only 1000 calories per day. To make this happen, there should be a controlled intake of a solid diet, whereas the dieter must consume green juices about 3 times a day. To minimize the calorie intake, rely more on fresh fruits and vegetables, and take small meals 2 times a day. Stay focused and stay determined, as these first three days can be the hardest, but you will get through them eventually

The remaining 4 days of this first phase of the Sirtfood diet introduces a bit of relaxation in the calorie restriction. During these days, the dieter can have 1500 calories per day. This means that they can introduce more solid food into the diet.

PHASE II of Sirtfood Diet

Phase II of the sirtfood diet can last for the next 14 days. If a dieter successfully completes the first phase of this diet plan, the second phase gets much easier. It is more about the maintenance of the weight and the new dietary regime. In this phase, there are no calorie restrictions in place, but the dieter must increase his sirtfood intake. Add as much sirtfood to your breakfast, lunch, dinner, and desserts as you can. The recipes in this cookbook will help you find a perfect combination of sirtfood ingredients for every meal. During these 14 days, the dieter can now decrease their daily green juice intake to two times per day.

Though there are no restrictions on calorie intake, the dieter must continue eating healthy and according to the calorie needs of the body.

Note: A little physical activity, along with this diet, is essential to losing weight in the given time. Hitting the gym every now and then is not necessary, only carry out light and regular 15-minute exercises which could help stimulate your metabolism and allow your body to better adapt to the new and healthy diet. That may include yoga, stretching exercises, swimming, cycling, playing outdoor sports, walking, jogging, etc.

SIRTFOOD GREEN JUICE

The sirtfood diet is incomplete without green juices. It provides all the antioxidants and Sirtuin activators that we need to stimulate sirtuin activity in our body. But why do we need green juices when you easily eat other sirtfood? Well, during the first phase of the sirtfood diet, the dieter needs to maintain calorie intake from 1000 to 1500 calories a day. Green juices are those low-calorie or zero-calorie drinks which do not add many calories to the diet, but they do add a lot of antioxidants and Sirtuin activators. That's why green juice is considered an essential part of this Sirtfood diet. In the first phase, green juices must be consumed 3 times per day, and then intake of green juices can be reduced to 2 times per day during the second phase.

The following are some of the main ingredients that you can regularly use to make your green juices:

- kale
- rocket
- parsley
- celery sticks
- green apple
- ginger
- lemon juice
- Matcha green tea

Extra-virgin olive oil

Extra virgin olive oil is mandatory in a daily diet plan. Olive oil itself has so many health advantages that's why we should consume it regularly. We can use it in several different ways, from seasoning the salads to searing the meat, and vegetables.

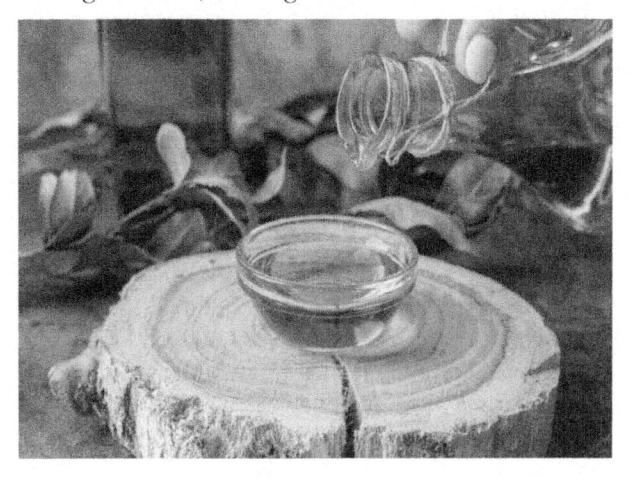

Rocket or Arugula

These dark green leaves are commonly used in salads, and they are a rich source of polyphenols. You can practically add arugula to every salad recipe by making a bowl of side salad or serve the meal with seasoned arugula leaves on the side.

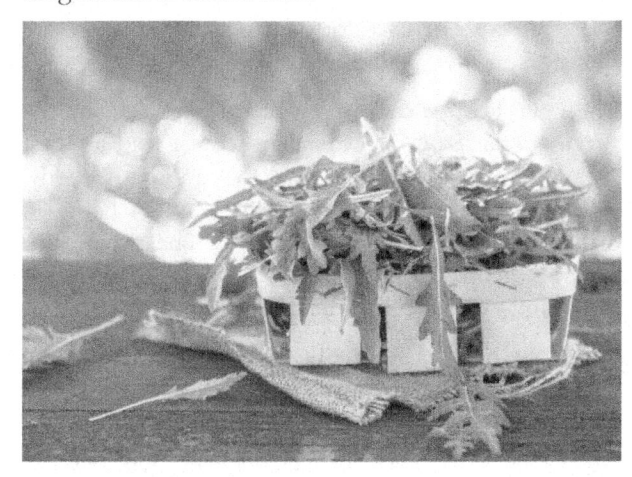

Soy

You can consume soybeans and its varieties in many ways. Soy milk that can be added to diet or tofu can also be used in many ways, which is made up of processed soybeans. Soy-based products are easily available in the market. You can use them all, but these products must be free from sweeteners, additives, and preservatives. In fact, the vegan feta cheese, which is recommended for every vegan menu, is also made with tofu, which is processed from soy.

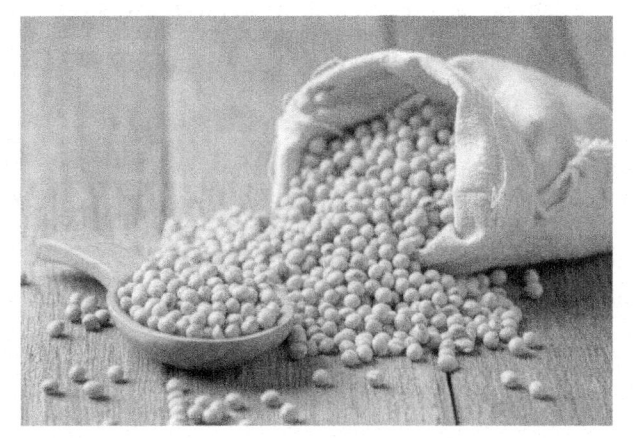

Strawberries

Strawberries are bright red, juicy, and sweet. They're an excellent source of vitamin C and manganese and also contain decent amounts of folate and potassium. Strawberries are very rich in antioxidants and plant compounds, which may have benefits for heart health and blood sugar control. They are used for nice garnishing for every dessert. You can easily increase your sirtfood intake by adding a handful of whole or sliced strawberries to a bowl of buckwheat porridge or enjoying some buckwheat pancake.

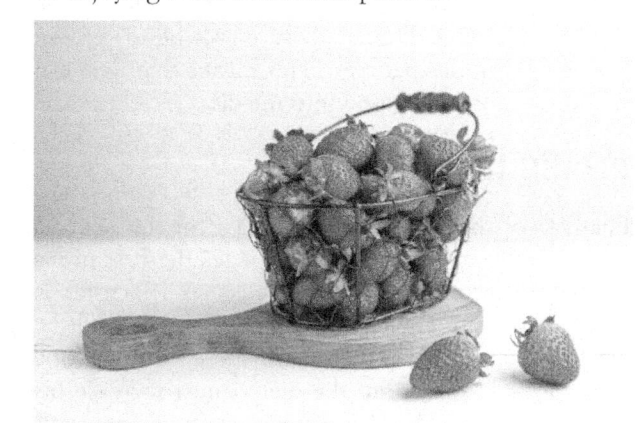

Kale

Kale being rich leafy greens can add the much-needed sirtuins to daily meals. The best thing is that kale can be consumed in many ways; chopped leaves can be consumed in morning omelet, or can be consumed in refreshing green juice, or make a salad. Kale can be added to soups, stews, or can be served with meat or steaks with sautéed kale.

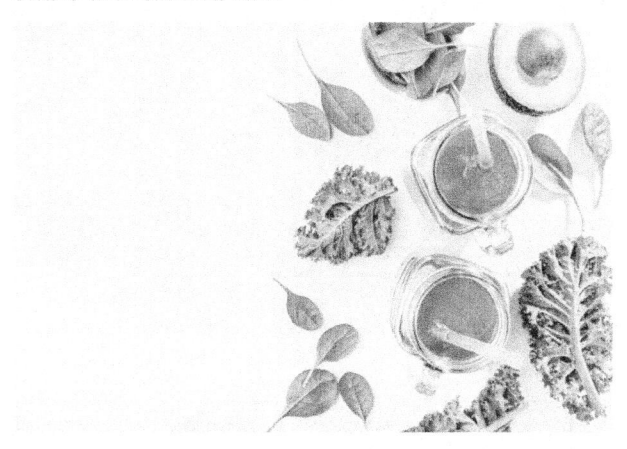

Blueberries

Blueberries are a little reservoir of nutrients; they are loaded with micronutrients, and they can increase your Sirtuin intake up to many folds. Blueberries can be consumed in many ways, like smoothies, juices, with morning porridges, and they can also be added to the desserts like cakes, muffins, etc.

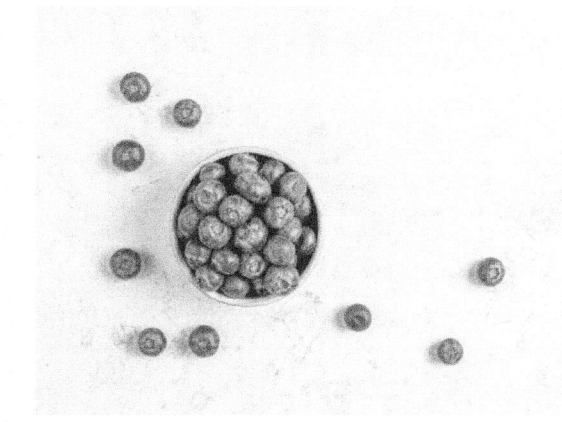

Red Wine

Red wine is another good Sirtfood as it is rich in antioxidants, and it is also known for its anti-inflammatory effects.

You can consume a glass of red wine every other day on a sirtfood diet, or some amount of red wine can be added to daily food.

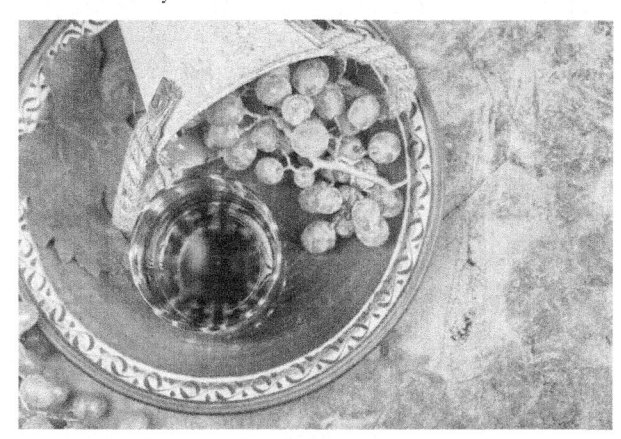

Green Tea

Green tea is full of antioxidants, and it can protect the cells from damage during the healing process. Green tea contains lots of phytonutrients that are anti-inflammatory, that are good for digestion, and they help in fat burning in the body. Green tea can help to weight loss when taken in combination with other Sirtuin-rich ingredients.

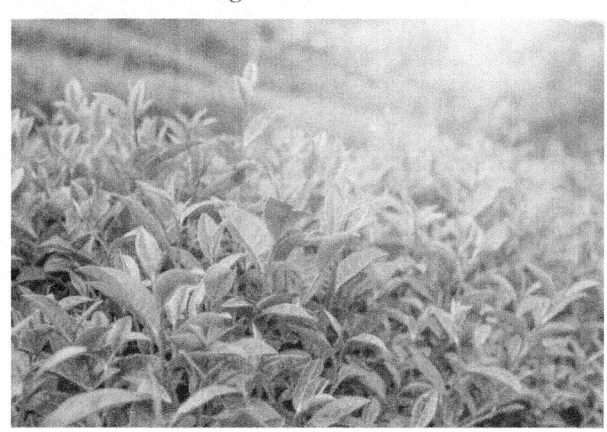

Turmeric

Turmeric is an Indian spice that is commonly used in Indian cuisine. It is already known for its wide-ranging healing effects. You can increase your antioxidant intake by adding ground or fresh turmeric to your diet.

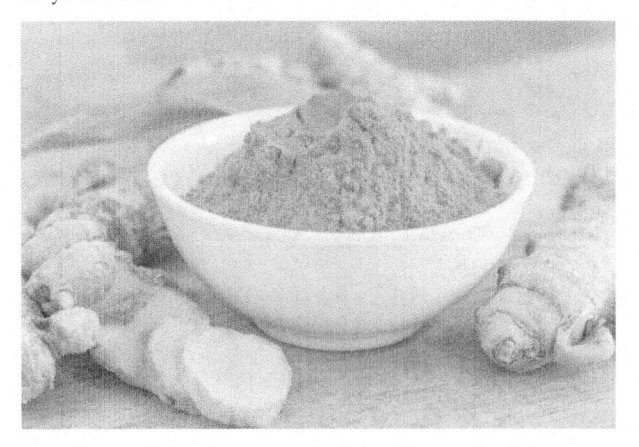

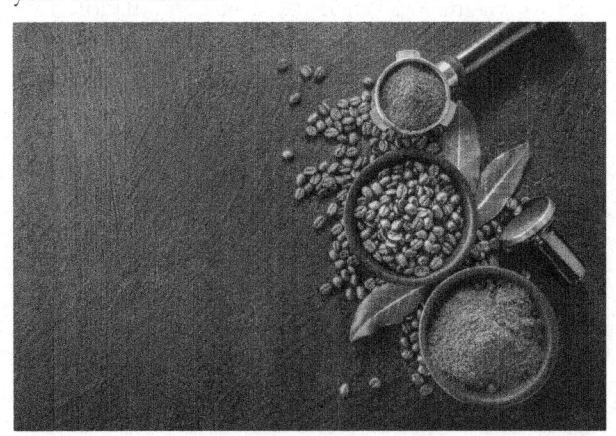

Onions

Onion can be used frequently in your meals is another sirtfood item that can increase your polyphenol intake. Onions can be added to salads, soups, stews, snacks, curries, etc.

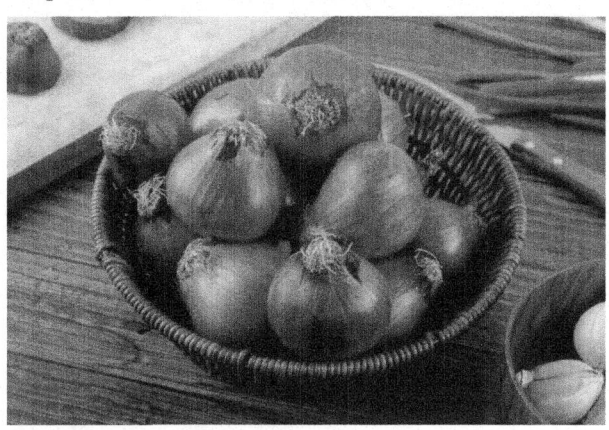

Coffee

Coffee is very rich in antioxidants — including polyphenols and hydrocinnamic acids — that may improve health and reduce your risk of several diseases. You can enjoy a cup of coffee and can increase. That's right, coffee beans also come up with those polyphenols which can stimulate and activate your Sirtuin intake.

Walnuts

Walnuts have the highest contents of antioxidants. Walnuts contribute significantly to the dietary intake of antioxidants. Add walnut, chopped, or whole to desserts like in muffins, bread, cakes, or buckwheat porridges on your sirtfood diet. Walnuts also have essential oils, minerals, and vitamins.

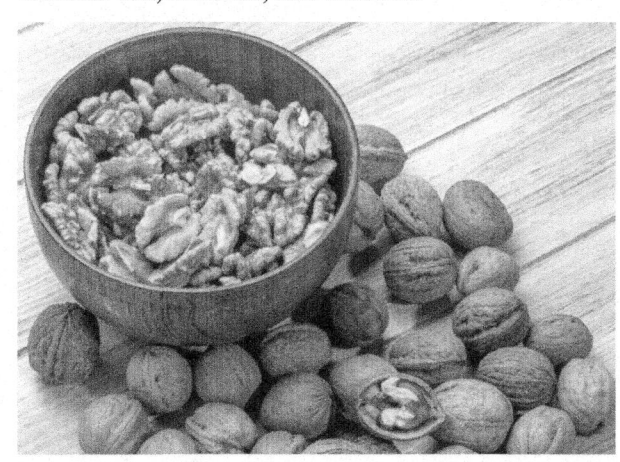

Buckwheat

Buckwheat is a perfect food to substitute wheat-based meals on your sirtfood diet. Buckwheat flour can be used to make bread, pancakes, tortillas, cakes, and other baked goods. Buckwheat groats can also be cooked to make the morning porridges. Buckwheat groats can also be added to the soups, stews, and some salads. Other Sirtuin-rich ingredients like strawberries, Medjool dates, or dark chocolate to a bowl of buckwheat porridge to make it a perfect morning meal.

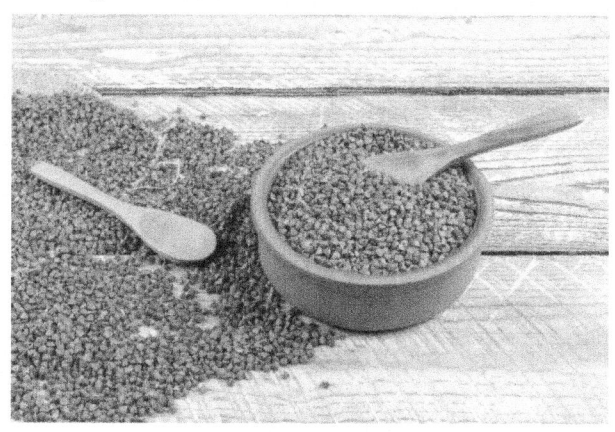

Parsley

Parsley leaves are famous for their distinctive aroma and added to most of the recipes to add a refreshing taste. They can also be used to garnish your meals or add them to your sirtfood green juices.

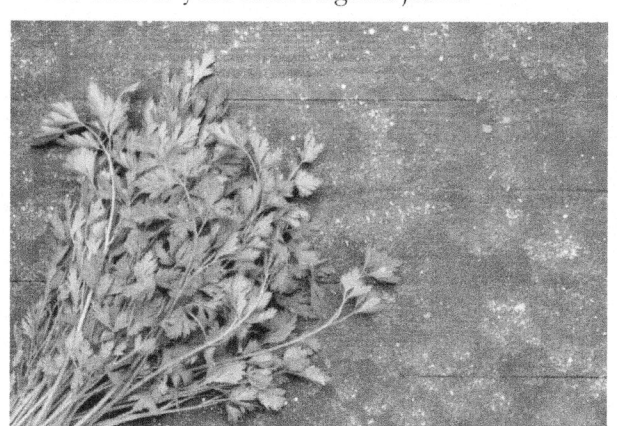

Chili

The antioxidant content of mature chili peppers is much higher than that of immature peppers. Chili peppers are rich in antioxidants that are linked to various health benefits. Chilies, whether green or red, are healthy for the sirtfood diet, and you can use them in a small amount in your routine meals.

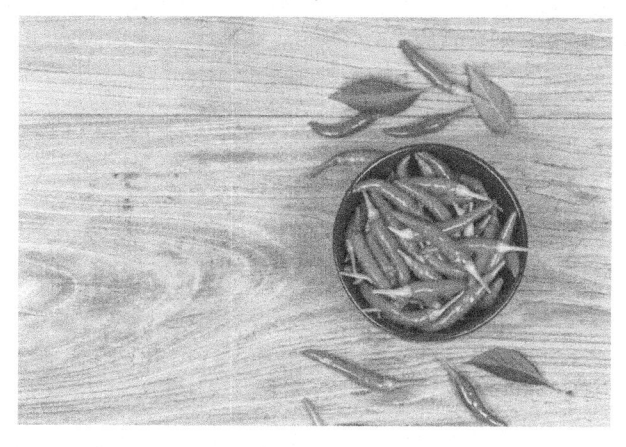

Medjool Dates

Medjool dates are also a rich source of antioxidants that help to fight damage caused by unstable molecules called free radicals. They contained carotenoid and phenolic acid antioxidants; both have beneficial effects on heart health. Those are just the things we need for this sirtfood diet. Medjool dates can be used in smoothies, desserts, and porridges. Adding whole or chopped Medjool dates to the desserts and breakfast provides sweetness without the use of other sweeteners.

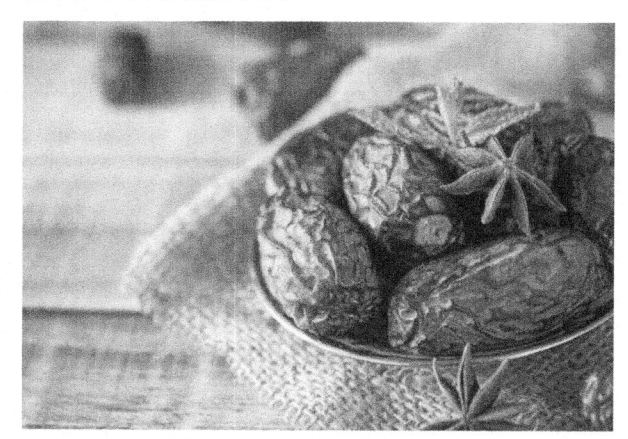

Celery

Celery is a great source of important antioxidants. Celery contains vitamin C, beta carotene, and flavonoids, but there are at least 12 additional kinds of antioxidant nutrients found in a single stalk. It can be consumed on this diet due to its high Sirtuin content. Celery is used in soups, broths, stews, smoothies, and salads for the best taste.

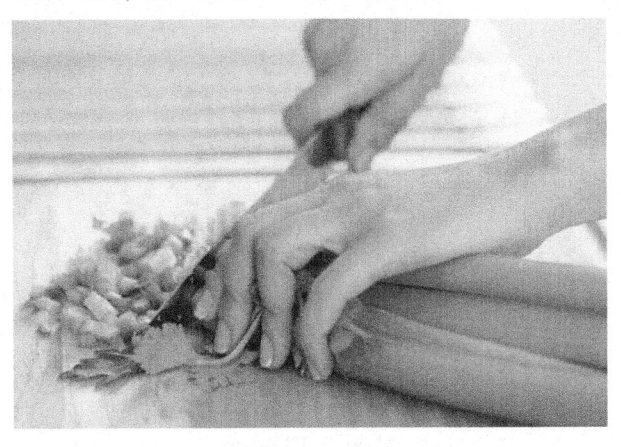

Lovage

Lovage leaves can be used in soups, stews, stir-fries, stocks, and other poultry or meat dishes. You can consume lovage to any of your green juices in sirtrfood diet. It is commonly known as sea parsley, the lovage leaves actually have a celery-like flavor.

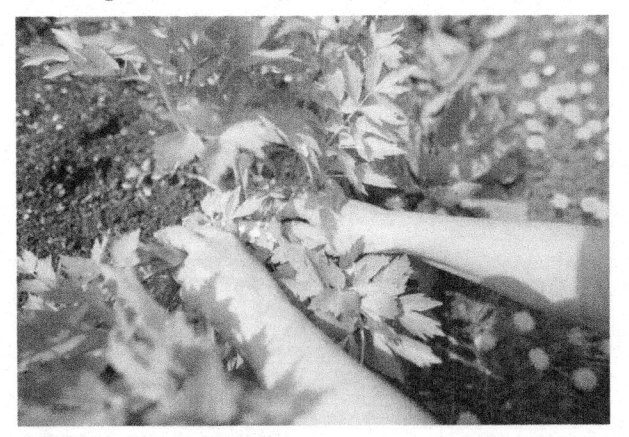

Dark Chocolate

Dark chocolate is another rich source of sirtuins activators, and it also contains lots of flavonoids that are good for the heart, digestion, and mental health of a person. The use of dark chocolate in the diet is a good way to fight all the sugar cravings, and it can be in a variety of ways in desserts. Dark chocolate mousse, chocolate muffins, chocolate balls can be consumed as a dessert.

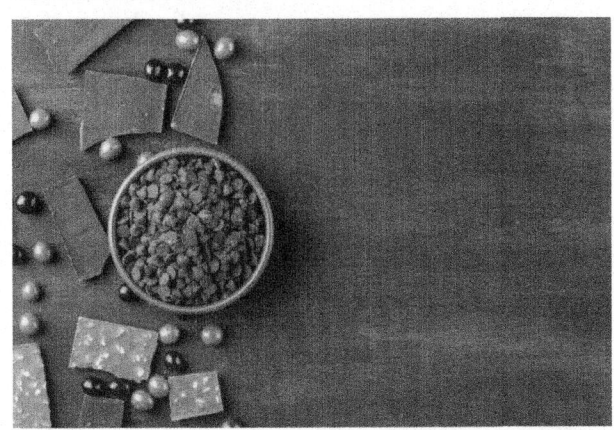

Foods to Avoid Having on the Sirtfood Diet

The sirtfood diet dose not restrictive to stop eating anything, but it demands the intake of more healthy food to maintain the calorie restriction and dieter must avoid having too much sugar, high carbs snacks, and processed food and replace them with healthier options like fresh or frozen fruits, vegetables and juices.

Sirtfood Diet for Vegans

Sirtfood diet can be both vegan and non-vegan. You can strictly keep your sirtfood diet vegan by avoiding meat, dairy, and other animal-based products. Add tofu, seitan, tempeh, vegan cheese, nut-based milk to replace the animal-based ingredients in your sirtfood diet.

Sirtfood diet and diabetics

Diabetics can use this diet if their health expert approves of this new dietary guideline. They need to be careful, as the first phase of this diet requires intense calorie restrictions, which can be dangerous for diabetic patients. So, they must consult their doctor and dietician while adopting this diet.

Sirtfood diet and PCOS

Sirtfood diet can help to relieve the symptoms of polycystic ovarian syndrome. Obesity is the major factor contributing to or aggravating the symptoms of PCOS, and by dealing with obesity, the sirtfood diet helps relieve its symptoms.

Sirtfood diet & Alcohol

Alcohol is not allowed during the first phase of the sirtfood diet; you can consume only water, green juices, green tea, and other low calories fruit juices instead. In the second phase, you have an intake of red wine or it can be added to your food, which only contains 14-15 percent of alcoholic content.

Sirtfood Diet & Oats

There is no harm in having oats on the sirtfood diet. However, you can take buckwheat groats and flakes instead of oats alternative. You can make porridge, pancakes, cakes, muffins, biscuits, and a variety of other desserts and snacks using buckwheat flour, which is a healthy sirtfood.

Sirtfood Diet

28 - Days Meal Plan

WEEK-1 SIRTFOOD MEAL PLAN

	MONDAY	TUESDAY	WEDNESDAY	THURSDAY	FRIDAY	SATURDAY	SUNDAY
BREAKFAST	Parsley Green Juice	Spinach & Apple Juice	Parsley Creamy Juice	Cilantro & Lettuce Juice	Cucumber Creamy Juice	Kale & Kiwi Juice	Broccoli Green Juice
LUNCH	Baked Green Beans	Steamed Broccoli with Olive Tahini	One-Pot Broccoli and Tofu	Tofu Wrap	Buffalo Broccoli Wings	Creamy Spinach Curry	Broccoli Pizza Pie
MIDDAY SNACK	Rocket Green Juice	Lettuce Green Juice	Broccoli Lime Juice	Fluffy avocado Juice	Broccoli Green Juice	Rocket Green Juice	Swiss Chard Green Juice
DINNER	Cilantro & Lettuce Juice	Cucumber Creamy Juice	Kale & Kiwi Juice	Broccoli Green Juice	Swiss Chard Green Juice	Kale Green Juice	Arugula leaves Juice

WEEK-2 SIRTFOOD MEAL PLAN

	MONDAY	TUESDAY	WEDNESDAY	THURSDAY	FRIDAY	SATURDAY	SUNDAY
Morning Juice	Berries Green Juice	Fluffy avocado Juice	Broccoli Green Juice	Rocket Green Juice	Swiss Chard Green Juice	Kale Green Juice	Arugula leaves Juice
Breakfast	Spinach Porridge	Italian Spinach Tofu Omelet	Tofu & Arugula Toast	Breakfast Tofu Scramble	Breakfast Tofu Waffles	Savory Buckwheat Porridge	French Toast with Berries
LUNCH	Steamed Kale with Walnuts	Hot & Spicy Tofu & Kale	Tofu, Broccoli & Soba Noodles	Broccoli Falafel	Creamy Kale Stew	Tofu with Buckwheat	Stir Fried Asparagus
DINNER	Parsley Creamy Juice	Cilantro & Lettuce Juice	Cucumber Creamy Juice	Kale & Kiwi Juice	Rocket Green Juice	Lettuce Green Juice	Broccoli Lime Juice

WEEK-3 SIRTFOOD MEAL PLAN

	Monday	Tuesday	Wednesday	Thursday	Friday	Saturday	Sunday
Morning Juice	Kale, Celery & Pear Juice	Green Fruit Juice	Spinach & Apple Juice	Parsley Green Juice	Cilantro & Lettuce Juice	Mix Green Juice	Rosemary Green Juice
Breakfast	Toast with Caramelized Apple	Acai Berry Smoothie Bowl	Morning Parfait	Spinach Muffins	Buckwheat Waffles	Chocolate Granola	Buckwheat Porridge with berries
Lunch	Broccoli Olives Pizza	Spicy Spinach Fillet	Wilted Spinach with Onion	Spinach & Tofu Curry	Hot & Sour Spinach	Tofu Power Bowls	Superfood Bibimbap with Crispy Tofu
Dinner	**Spinach Soup**	Hot & Sour Soup	Simple Tofu Quiche	Cauliflower Mac 'n' Cheese	Chicken Stew	Salmon & Lentils	Tofu with Chickpeas & Kale

WEEK-4 SIRTFOOD MEAL PLAN

	MONDAY	TUESDAY	WEDNESDAY	THURSDAY	FRIDAY	SATURDAY	SUNDAY
Morning Juice	Cucumber Creamy Juice	Broccoli Green Juice	Berries Green Juice	Berries Green Juice	Green Juice Recipe	Healthy Green Juice with Lemon	Tomato-Kale Gazpacho Smoothie
Breakfast	Berries Pancakes	Chocolate Pancakes	Tofu & Spinach Muffins	Tofu & Berries Waffles	Tofu & Berries Waffles	Tofu & Kale Toast	Buckwheat Pancakes
LUNCH	Spicy Tofu Kale Wraps	Tofu Burritos	Baked Chicken with Salad	Lamb Chops with Salad	Flank Steak with Salad	Glazed Flank Steak	Stir-Fried Asparagus
DINNER	Buckwheat Noodles with Beef	Chicken Breast with Asparagus	Buckwheat Noodles with Shrimp	Slow Cooker Salmon & walnut Soup	Salmon with Pesto & Beans	Mushrooms & Kale Stew	Stir-Fried Shrimp & Kale
Snacks	Beet Root & Kale Hummus	Healthy Berries Smoothie Bowl	Chicken Snacks	Tofu & Blueberries Pie	Sirtfood Dates Bites	Dark Chocolate Cookies	Cinnamon Chocolate Bites

Made in the USA
Monee, IL
05 July 2021